What Is It and How Did I Get It? Early Stage Chronic Kidney Disease

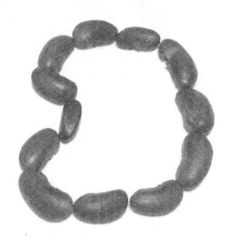

Gail Rae

First published by Dog Ear Publishing
4010 W. 86th Street, Ste H
Indianapolis, IN 46268
www.dogearpublishing.net

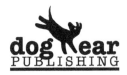

ISBN: 978-145750-214-9

This book is printed on acid-free paper.

Printed in the United States of America

Table of Contents

Disclaimer

I am not a doctor, nor do I pretend to be one. All I am is a patient, one who was very confused when first diagnosed. While I fully intend to share what I've learned since then, that is my only intent. I can neither prescribe, nor be the authority on all things medical. Speak to your doctor when you need advice, but take some comfort from knowing you are not alone in needing some help along the way.

Note: As you read this book, you'll notice certain words written in bold letters the first time they're used. These are the words you'll find explained in the glossary at the back of the book.

Acknowledgements

Paul Garwood, better known as "Bear," willingly accepted all things **renal** as part of me: exercise, diet, tests, lots and lots of doctors' appointments. How lucky I am to have met you just before this journey began, my love. My children, Nima Beckie and Abby Wegerski, gave me the freedom to become a writer when they really should have been selfish little things, but weren't. You are my blessings. My chosen sister, Cheryl Vincent, has spent most of her time reminding me to take care of myself while we explored how much trouble we could get into together. I guess angels do exist.

CHAPTER 1:

Introduction

This book is titled *What Is It and How Did I Get It?* Those were the first questions I blurted when I was told there was even a chance of having a kidney disease. I'd never heard of this. We were a family that had cancer problems, not kidney problems. I knew the kidneys were some kind of internal organs, but that's all I knew about them. **Chronic Kidney Disease**? I was mystified. I did realize that **chronic** is not **acute**. It means long term, whereas acute usually means quick onset and short duration. So, I had a progressive something or other that affected my kidneys.

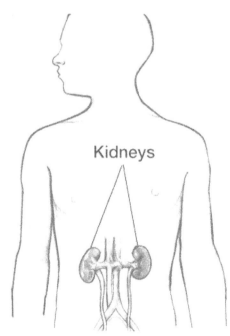

Kidneys

Later, I learned that the kidneys were two reddish brown organs which

National Institute of Diabetes and Digestive and Kidney Diseases, National Institutes of Health.

- 1 -

lay on the muscles of the back on either side of your spine above hipbone level and below the diaphragm, just as the diagram on the previous page shows. Some have compared their size to that of a clenched fist or a large computer mouse, and the right one lies lower than the left since the liver is on that side.

Ingested food and liquid are digested in the stomach and bowels, and then absorbed in the blood. A renal artery carries the blood, waste and water to the kidneys while a renal vein carries the filtered and sieved waste from the kidneys.

Yes the kidneys are bean shaped. I wondered if the kidneys were named for the beans or vice versa, but didn't wonder enough to research it. There were so many, more important issues to research at this point in my life.

I remembered hearing somewhere that if one kidney is damaged the other could sustain a person. I researched that. It was true. They are hardworking organs, too. They filter as many as 200 quarts of blood per day to rid us of roughly two quarts of waste and extra water.

These two organs, the master chemists of our bodies, have several functions: regulating the fluid balance in the body, providing vital **hormones**, producing **erythropoietin**, and producing the **renin** that regulates blood pressure. This is why **CKD** patients need to be careful about sodium, **potassium**, chloride, **calcium**, magnesium, and phosphates. Your nutritionist may not even mention magnesium to you since this constitutes only 1% of extra cellular fluid. Additional important jobs of the kidneys are removing liquid waste from your body and balancing the minerals in the body. The two liquid waste products are urea which has been broken down from **protein** by the digestive system and creatinine which is a byproduct of muscle activity.

The problem with unregulated minerals, such as sodium and potassium, is that these minerals are needed to remain healthy but too much in the bloodstream becomes toxic. The kidneys remove these toxins and change them into urine that enters the bladder via the **ureter**. Picture a front view of your internal organs. You see the ribs, below them the kidneys, then the ureter above the bladder. Below the bladder is the urethra, the passage to the outside of your body. This is, of course, a highly simplified explanation. The toxins would build up and poison you if the kidneys were damaged. I immediately began to wonder if that held true if you had CKD, too.

My new family doctor explained that one of my blood test results indicated CKD might be something I had, but a specialist was needed to deal with this. Then she showed me the Estimated **GFR** on my tri-monthly blood test results and asked me how long it had been this low. I looked at her blankly. Estimated GFR? Low? How long? How should I know? My former doctor's Physician's Assistant [**P.A.**] had always interpreted these blood tests for liver function. I'd been having these tests for quite a while since I was taking a medication that just might affect the liver somewhere down the line. That's the liver, not the kidneys. No one had ever used the term estimated GFR with me before.

Wait a minute, why hadn't my previous doctor told me about the possible problem, I demanded. This thorough physician quickly explained that these results didn't mean I HAD this disease, just that I might. The results might mean nothing, but they had to be explored. I later realized that my reaction was almost text book: shocked, confused, angry and disbelieving. And just like everyone else who is given a **nephrology** appointment very quickly, I figured out that this was serious.

As soon as my appointment ended, I raced to my home office where I had copies of my laboratory [**lab**] work from the previous doctor. Looking at the lab reports which covered a seven month period, I found the first report mentioned not being able to estimate the GFR since no age or gender had been provided [more on that in Chapter 7]. That made no sense to me at the time. Six months later the estimated GFR had been 49 and, when retested one month after that, it was 60. Since there are one to two million neprhons in each kidney, a decrease in their function may not be noticed until the early stages of CKD. It looked like that's what happened to me.

I still didn't understand this, so I called the P.A. I'd formerly dealt with who explained that the estimated GFR of 49 was troublesome enough to order another test a month later. The re-test test showed an estimated GFR of 60 which was considered borderline for Chronic Kidney Disease [CKD]. But what was a GFR? And what did these numbers mean?

I could see the logic based on the higher and lower numbers, but I didn't grasp that this could be happening to me, and I didn't know anything about it. I'd always been so in tune with my body that I could tell when I was becoming ill before any symptoms showed up (oddly enough, my curly hair would become temporarily straight if I were incubating some illness or other), but not this time. I was involved with organic and healthy eating, with herbal supplements to strengthen my body, but they seemed to be doing me no good in this case. I danced vigorously several times a week for exercise, yet I was still having some kind of medical problem.

Further confusing the issue is the fact that the kidneys simply work harder during the early stages of CKD, so patients feel no symptoms. Sufferers don't start to feel ill until kidney function is as low as 10%. That could take a long time, maybe 10 years. My **nephrologist** suggested that would be 20 years for me since he suspected the cause of my disease to be old age and that my kidney function would probably decrease only ½% a year. I didn't like being called old, but I'd take it if it meant I would have such a long time without dialysis ahead of me.

There's also a theory that keeping the blood pressure under control can delay dialysis. After all, the kidneys do release renin. I'd been on an **ACE inhibitor** for over 20 years, not knowing that this could also slow the progression of my CKD. I strive for a blood pressure reading of 130/80 or lower. Although, the medication apparently has done too good a job of this since I'm presently dealing with LOW blood pressure.

Through my research, I began to understand what high blood pressure [**HPB**] has to do with renal disease. HPB can damage small blood vessels in the kidneys to the point that they cannot filter the waste from the blood as effectively as they should. Nephrologists may prescribe HBP medication to prevent your CKD from getting worse since these medications reduce the amount of protein in your urine. Not too surprisingly, most CKD related deaths are caused by cardiovascular problems.

What especially troubled me is that even a small amount of kidney function decline can double the risk for cardiovascular problems. It's been over two years for me, but I still have trouble understanding that I am at risk for a heart attack or stroke. But what makes me angry is that now that I have CKD, my children have an increased risk of developing it as well.

I called and e-mailed family members, both closely and distantly related. I found HBP, high **cholesterol**, cancerous and **benign** tumors and Parkinson's disease in the family, but nothing that affected the kidneys. This became more and more puzzling, to say nothing of the panic I started to feel.

Didn't people die from kidney disease? My younger daughter had just become engaged, and my older one lived across the country from me. How could I interrupt their lives with the news of another medical complication? And, frankly, I just plain didn't want to die which I thought was going to happen soon. I was frightened, so I started doing what I usually did when I was in a spot: research – something no one in a panic state should have to do since the panic colors your interpretation of the material.

Meanwhile, my new family physician helped me find a specialist who was covered by my insurance. I lived in Arizona but had a New York based insurance company, so I needed the help. I see the specialist twice a year. It could have cost me hundreds of dollars each visit, but with the insurance I was only responsible for the minimal co-pay. This is why it's important to find a nephrologist on your medical insurance plan.

As it turned out, I hadn't even known that this specialist was called a nephrologist, despite my English teacher knowledge of Greek [nephros] & Latin [renes] roots. I began to wonder how my education could help me deal with this serious disease, if it could at all. Maybe my computer skills were more important here.

Asking the doctor questions wouldn't help me, because I didn't know what to ask at this point. Although I intended to comply with his office's request that I bring either the medications I took or a list of them with their specific names, dosages and the frequency of taking them as well as a list of all the natural or alternative medications I took. I intended to also bring a list of questions with me; I knew that being nervous would cause all those pertinent questions to fly right out of my mind.

I think I would have offered my symptoms too, but I didn't have any that I could recognize. I'd already had my medical history faxed to the nephrologist, and I didn't think x-rays of my previously broken bones would be of any help, so I didn't bring them. If you do have some pertinent film such a Magnetic Resonance Image [**MRI**] or Computerized Axial Tomography Scan [**CAT scan**], it would be a good idea to bring it with you on that first visit. This is a good place to mention that intravenous dye sometimes used with an MRI or a CAT scan for contrast is not a good idea with CKD, especially if the CKD is Stage 3 or higher. Another kind of dye, ingested dye, however, remains in your intestines nowhere near your kidneys, so that doesn't present a problem. One thing I was absolutely sure I would be doing is taking notes, so I could review them at home, and maybe even ask for a sketch of where the kidneys were if it still wasn't clear to me after it was explained.

Nearly 30 million people in the U.S. have CKD or **nephropathy** and that number was projected to increase by 7% each year. That's 13% of our country's population. Now, I was one of them. 40% of all this kidney failure was caused by suffering diabetes for a decade or more. My CKD wasn't.

Before my first appointment with the nephrologist, I collected and read everything I could about CKD from the internet. Some of it was contradictory, some of it was really old, some of it was too scientific, some of it seemed to be right on the mark, but all of it was confusing no matter how simplistically it was written. I had no frame of reference and needed help interpreting what I was reading.

I knew I would ask the nephrologist for some books that were neither too scientific nor too simplistic. That's how I learned: I read books even with the internet available to me. Sometimes, as in this case, I learned by writing a book about the subject.

So I confused myself many times over until I saw this specialist. He did explain what CKD was and how I might have gotten it, but so quickly that – again - I couldn't understand it all. He knew his stuff, that was abundantly clear, but his style was paternalistic while I needed a doctor who was interested in working with me rather than unilaterally taking care of me. It's a small distinction, and I mean no disrespect to my first nephrologist. I just needed a different style of doctoring.

Prior to having this disease sneak up on me, I might have been perfectly content with his style. Now I was nervous that my body wasn't telling me everything, and I wanted an active role in monitoring it. I wanted a doctor who would talk to me about every inconsistency in my tests, who would ask me questions that would open a discussion about my condition. I wanted a partner, but one who had far more information than I did about CKD.

Luckily, there was another doctor in the same practice that one of the nurses thought I might be able to work with. She was right. This nephrologist had the same information as the first one, but his style was more open to partnership with the patient rather than taking the sole responsibility for the care of the patient. That's what I'd been looking for.

Many patients prefer the paternalistic type of doctoring, and there is no shame in that. It's almost like a marriage in that you choose each other based on your particular needs. The first nephrologist's style and mine didn't match at this point in my medical history although they might have just a few months before when there hadn't been anything seriously amiss in my body.

By this time, although I still had so much to learn, I'd already been to see the nutritionist associated with the practice. She had started to teach me about potassium, sodium, **phosphorous** and food units. The sodium information was familiar to me since I had HPB, but the rest was an eye opener. She also gave me something magical: a printed copy of the renal diet. Here was something I could relate to, something I could turn to constantly to look up whatever I wasn't sure about, something I could carry with me as my security blanket until I got a handle on just what this CKD was and how to deal with it.

This second nephrologist explained, and in all honesty I do believe the first one mentioned this too, that they didn't really know how I got this disease which is so prevalent that more than 25% of **Medicare** payments, roughly 42 billion dollars, went towards its treatment. In fact, the U.S. has the highest rate of CKD with 210 people per million having it, and two thirds of those cases caused by diabetes or HBP.

The theory was that it was associated with the HBP I'd had for over 20 years since I didn't have any of the other presumed causes: diabetes, years of almost daily use of non-steroidal anti-inflammatories [Advil, Aleve, Motrin, Tylenol, Ibuprofen, etc.] long time or high dosage use of Lithium, or multiple corrective surgeries for urinary drainage as a child. Nor was I a Native American, Alaskan Native, Hispanic, Pacific Islander or Afro-American, ethnic groups that have a 15 to 17% higher occurrence of CKD. So I didn't have a higher susceptibility to CKD, except for the fact that I was over 50, another group that is more affected by CKD.

I wasn't even male, which might have slightly raised my chances for contracting this disease. I'd never had gout, the disease in which uric acid usually excreted in the urine goes into the blood instead, so that couldn't be the cause. I hadn't developed high levels of triglycerides along with low levels of HDL cholesterol, so that was out as a possible predictor of my CKD.

All my nephrologist and I could look at was the **hypertension** and my age although the age factor wasn't mentioned until two years into my disease. That was two years during which I'd been driving myself slightly batty trying to figure out why I got this disease. Obesity is sometimes suspect since it can lead to diabetes, one of the causes of CKD. But, I didn't have any indications of diabetes, despite my weight, not even high blood sugar.

My problem in understanding this was that my hypertension had been controlled for 20 years. How could a controlled problem cause another problem? There seemed to be no answer. Recently, I've even come across a theory that a potassium deficiency could also be a cause.

At a subsequent nephrologist visit, it was explained that this disease could also be age related since the number of **nephrons** decrease as you age, and that I'd continue to lose about 1/2% of my kidney function each year. That made more sense to me than successfully treated hypertension causing it. You age, your kidneys age.

The number of nephrons decreases, as does the amount of kidney tissue. If the blood vessels supplying the kidneys harden, it will take the kidneys longer to filter your blood. The formerly elastic tissue of the bladder wall is replaced with tough, fibrous tissue so that the bladder is less stretchable. When the muscles weaken, you may not empty your bladder completely.

Oh boy, did I have a lot to look forward to, especially if this process of kidney deterioration had already started. Of course, the cause still can't be pinpointed, but I liked the idea that dialysis wouldn't be entering the picture for at least 20 years according to the expected kidney function percentage for the next 20 years. As I researched, I began to realize that the thought of dialysis – not the disease itself – was what had been frightening and repulsing me. I needed to understand that I could work toward keeping dialysis at bay for a couple of decades.

As for what CKD is, I was told that it's a slowly decreasing function of the kidneys. Of course, then I needed to see a chart of where the kidneys are and an explanation of what they did. No wonder my research was confusing. CKD wasn't any of the kidney diseases I'd uncovered on the internet. It was simple CKD which was also known as Chronic Renal Insufficiency or Chronic Renal Failure. What horrified me was that this disease doesn't stop or get better. The best you could expect was to slow it down.

I vividly remember that when I was diagnosed, I blurted, "But my daughter's getting married!" I knew it was a very odd reaction to this serious announcement, but now several years later, I think it was my way of saying no to the disease. My life was just too full, too sweet, too important to me to stop it then. I had actually thought I was being given a death sentence.

That's what this book is about. I don't want anyone else to feel that way. Yes, your doctor and your nutritionist will help you understand the progression of your CKD and how to deal with it, but I want your path down that road to be a long, long one and understanding what's happening may help make this happen. After that first outburst, I hid my fears from everyone until I truly understood what was happening to me. It took too long by myself. I put myself through a long period of acting as if all was fine while, inside, I was constantly on the verge of panic. Not sharing your fears, your concerns with others will do that as I taught myself.

It's not that I couldn't get help from the nephrologist and nutritionist. It's that I couldn't even look at the disease long enough to formulate the questions I needed help answering. I needed a book like this one to help me, but there just weren't any available at the time. I didn't want a scientific explanation or a cookbook, not even a how to live with CKD book. I wanted a book written by someone with the disease who could give me the same information I'd get from a medical practitioner, but in a way that I could understand while I was frightened, shocked and pretty sad, too. My hope is that this is what my book will do for you.

CHAPTER 2:

Where It All Started

The Laboratory Report on the following pages is what my new primary care physician – a term I use interchangeably with family doctor or simply physician in this book - was looking at when she started asking me those questions I couldn't answer. I'd always accepted that copies of my quarterly blood tests were in my file at the doctor's office, and I'd be informed if there was a liver problem since I was taking these tests to monitor how my medication was affecting my liver function. I hadn't thought to ask about any other problems. I should have. You need to be aware of your lab reports, the findings and what they mean to you.

Look at the lab report on the next two pages. Above the results section was all the information needed to identify these as my tests. For my privacy, that of my primary care physician and the lab, this information has been blackened out. I did leave in the information that this was a **fasting** test, no eating or drinking after midnight the day before the blood and urine were collected. Each section is a different test with its own parts, so each part of each test is explained.

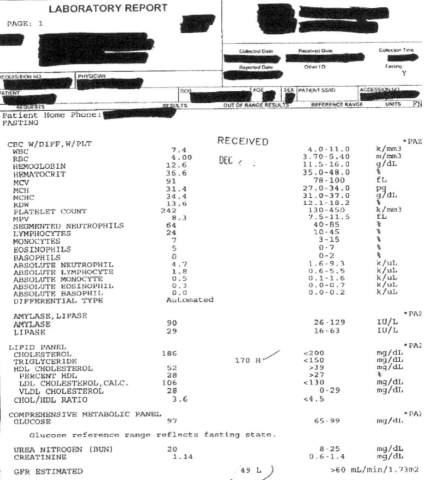

LABORATORY REPORT

PAGE: 1

| Collected Date | Received Date | Collection Time |
| Reported Date | Other I.D. | Fasting Y |

REQUISITION NO | PHYSICIAN

PATIENT | DOB | AGE | SEX | PATIENT SSID | ACCESSION (#)

REQUESTS | RESULTS | OUT OF RANGE RESULTS | REFERENCE RANGE | UNITS | PN

Patient Home Phone:
FASTING

RECEIVED

*PAZ

CBC W/DIFF,W/PLT				
WBC	7.4		4.0-11.0	k/mm3
RBC	4.00	DEC	3.70-5.40	m/mm3
HEMOGLOBIN	12.6		11.5-16.0	g/dL
HEMATOCRIT	36.6		35.0-48.0	%
MCV	91		78-100	fL
MCH	31.4		27.0-34.0	pg
MCHC	34.4		31.0-37.0	g/dL
RDW	13.6		12.1-18.2	%
PLATELET COUNT	242		130-450	k/mm3
MPV	8.3		7.5-11.5	fL
SEGMENTED NEUTROPHILS	64		40-85	%
LYMPHOCYTES	24		10-45	%
MONOCYTES	7		3-15	%
EOSINOPHILS	5		0-7	%
BASOPHILS	0		0-2	%
ABSOLUTE NEUTROPHIL	4.7		1.6-9.3	k/uL
ABSOLUTE LYMPHOCYTE	1.8		0.6-5.5	k/uL
ABSOLUTE MONOCYTE	0.5		0.1-1.6	k/uL
ABSOLUTE EOSINOPHIL	0.3		0.0-0.7	k/uL
ABSOLUTE BASOPHIL	0.0		0.0-0.2	k/uL
DIFFERENTIAL TYPE	Automated			

AMYLASE,LIPASE			*PA2
AMYLASE	90	26-129	IU/L
LIPASE	29	16-63	IU/L

LIPID PANEL				*PA2
CHOLESTEROL	186		<200	mg/dL
TRIGLYCERIDE		170 H	<150	mg/dL
HDL CHOLESTEROL	52		>39	mg/dL
PERCENT HDL	28		>27	%
LDL CHOLESTEROL,CALC.	106		<130	mg/dL
VLDL CHOLESTEROL	28		0-29	mg/dL
CHOL/HDL RATIO	3.6		<4.5	

COMPREHENSIVE METABOLIC PANEL			*PA2
GLUCOSE	97	65-99	mg/dL

Glucose reference range reflects fasting state.

UREA NITROGEN (BUN)	20		8-25	mg/dL
CREATININE	1.14		0.6-1.4	mg/dL
GFR ESTIMATED		49 L	>60 mL/min/1.73m2	

In African Americans, the calculated eGFR should be multiplied by
1.21.

The result >60 mL/min/1.73 m2 represents the upper limit of
reliability for the equation set up by the NKDEP. The reference range
for GFR is >90 mL/min/1.73 m2.

Note: eGFR calculation changed to IDMS-traceable equation effective
12/6/07.

BUN/CREAT RATIO	17.5		10.0-28.0	
SODIUM	142		135-145	mmol/L
POTASSIUM	3.7		3.5-5.2	mmol/L
CHLORIDE	102		96-110	mmol/L
CARBON DIOXIDE (CO2)	27		19-31	mmol/L
ANION GAP	13		4-18	
PROTEIN,TOTAL	7.0		6.0-8.0	g/dL
ALBUMIN	4.1		3.3-4.9	g/dL
GLOBULIN	2.9		2.1-3.9	g/dL
ALB/GLOB RATIO	1.4		1.0-2.0	
CALCIUM	9.7		8.4-10.6	mg/dL
ALKALINE PHOSPHATASE	81		39-170	IU/L
ALT	27		2-46	IU/L
AST	21		10-41	IU/L
BILIRUBIN, TOTAL	0.4		0.2-1.3	mg/dL

TSH W/REFLEX TO FREE T4   *PAZ

TSH	1.32		0.45-4.50	mU/L

UROGRAM W/RFLX MICRO and CULTURE   *PAZ

COLOR, URINE	Normal		Normal	
CLARITY, URINE	Clear		Clear	
SPECIFIC GRAVITY, URINE	1.019		1.005-1.030	
LEUKOCYTE ESTERASE		Moderate	Negative	
NITRITE, URINE QUAL	Negative		Negative	
pH, URINE	6.5		5.0-8.0	
BLOOD, URINE QUAL	Negative		Negative	
PROTEIN, URINE QUAL	Negative		Negative	mg/dL
GLUCOSE, URINE QUAL	Negative		Negative	mg/dL
KETONES, URINE QUAL	Negative		Negative	
UROBILINOGEN, URINE QUAL	Normal		Normal	EU/dL
BILE, URINE QUAL	Negative		Negative	

URINALYSIS, MICROSCOPIC   *PAZ

WBC, URINE	0-5		0-5	/hpf
RBC, URINE	None Seen		0-2	/hpf
EPITHELIAL CELLS, URINE	0-5		0-5	/hpf
BACTERIA, URINE	None Seen		None Seen	/hpf
HYALINE CASTS	None Seen		None Seen	/lpf

The Complete Blood Count [CBC] *with Diff,* */with Platelets* [Plt]

In plain English, this test measures the concentration of white blood cells [WBC], red blood cells [RBC], and platelets in the blood. All are important since each type of blood cell performs a different function:

1. The white blood cells make up your immune system. There are usually from 7,000 to 25,000 WBC in a drop of blood, but if you have an infection, that number rises since these are the infection fighting blood cells.
2. The red blood cells, also called erythrocytes, carry oxygen to the other cells in your body - so the higher the number here the better - and waste such as carbon dioxide from them. There are approximately five billion red blood cells – the mid sized cells – in a single drop of your blood.
3. The platelets deal with the blood's clotting ability by repairing leaks in your blood vessels. Normally, there are 150,000 to 350,000 platelets in one drop of blood.

Something I found interesting is that white blood cells are the largest, red ones smaller and platelets the smallest. Your blood is 60% plasma, which is a fluid so it transports elements to and from different parts of your body, and 40% blood cells.

Red blood cells usually live 120 days, but not with CKD, so they need to be replaced more often. You may not yet have heard of erythropoietin [EPO] from your nephrologist. This is the substance that travels from the kidneys via the blood to the bone marrow to trigger the manufacture of red blood cells. With CKD, less EPO is produced, so the bone marrow makes fewer red blood cells. That translates into **anemia**.

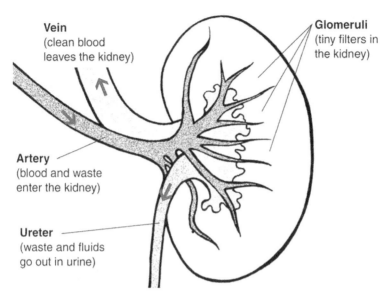

National Institute of Diabetes and Digestive and Kidney Diseases, National Institutes of Health.

"DIFF." describes each type of white blood cell or "differentiates" between them, and lists how many of each type of cell is present since each performs a different function. Lymphocytes, monocytes, basophils, eosinophils and neutrophils are different types of white blood cells. Notice that the neutrophils count refers to segmented, or mature, neutrophils.

The lower part of this list refers to the same elements as the previous part of the list, but is labeled "absolute" this time. Absolute means that a formula has been used to count each type of white blood cell.

The next set of results, although part of the same section of the test, is explained in table format to make it easier to understand.

Hemoglobin is the protein in red blood cells that carries oxygen from the lungs to the rest of the body. I didn't know it then but hemoglobin is important for CKD patients since a low hemoglobin count may indicate anemia.

Hematocrit reflects the percentage of blood volume that is made up of red blood cells, something else that is important to CKD patients.

Mean Corpuscular Volume [MCV] measures the average volume or size of individual red blood cells.

Mean Corpuscular Hemoglobin [MCH] measures the hemoglobin content of red blood cells.

Mean Corpuscular Hemoglobin Concentration [MCHC] measures the concentration of hemoglobin in the average red blood cell. (Low counts in any of these first five may be indicative of an anemia problem since all of them deal with the red blood cells.)

Mean Platelet Volume [MPV] describes the size of the platelets. Again a low count may be involved with anemia.

Red cell distribution width [RDW] is also important for CKD patients since it deals with different kinds of anemia.

My explanation of the tests is simplistic, but as you can see, none of the results in column 2 were out of range in column 3 according to the reference ranges in column 4. Good news for me. I've learned to watch hemoglobin and hematocrit. It'll be a little vague now, (all right, so it's a little boring, too) but both have to do with anemia which can be common in people with our disease. That word, anemia, kept coming up. Learning to read your own test results may help you prevent more severe anemia than that which you may already have.

Amylase and Lipase Enzymes
Amylase, Lipase

I glossed over the next section, too, since all was all right in my amylase - lipase world. Naturally, I had no idea what they were and didn't care since they weren't causing a problem for me. But then curiosity got the better of me, so I looked them up. Amylase is an enzyme that breaks starch down into sugar. The reading could be an indicator for diabetes, another cause of CKD. I already knew that this was not a cause of my CKD, but it was reassuring to see it right there in black and white.

Lipase is an enzyme necessary for the absorption and digestion of nutrients in the intestines. I wasn't sure why that was being tested until I researched a bit more and discovered that, even though an elevated level of this indicates a pancreatic problem, a mild increase of lipase in the blood could be an indication of kidney disease. Both tests were within range. More good news for me.

Lipid Panel

Then I hit the Lipid Panel. Uh-oh, look at the triglyceride test. All these years of taking medication to successfully control my cholesterol level and the triglyceride number was out of range. The quarterly blood tests I took were to monitor the cholesterol lowering medication's effect on my liver. I'd never had such a result in one of my blood tests before.

❖ The triglycerides are one of the bad cholesterols like low-density lipoprotein cholesterol [LDL] and could affect the heart and blood vessels by thickening them. I was a little confused as to what this had to do with CDK until I looked it up on my computer.

❖ Cholesterol is a natural substance in the body.

❖ High-density lipoprotein [HDL] is the good cholesterol that helps keep the LDL from lodging in your artery walls. A healthy level of HDL may also protect against heart attack and stroke.

❖ Triglycerides, another natural substance in the body, can also threaten to harden your coronary arteries. To be blunt, triglycerides are fat.

I recognized HDL cholesterol as the good cholesterol and LDL as the bad, but what was VLDL cholesterol? I discovered it's very low density lipoprotein, a transporter of cholesterol within the body just like HDL and LDL. Now I understood why this could be a problem for a CKD patient. Triglycerides and HDL had to be watched since they could compromise your heart health just as CKD could. The total cholesterol to HDL ratio [CHOL/HDL RATIO] is used as a predictor for heart disease although research scientists are not as convinced about its accuracy as doctors are.

Comprehensive Metabolic Panel

It got worse: while my glucose, urea nitrogen [BUN] and creatinine were within range, the Glomerular Filtration Rate [**GFR**] was certainly not above 60 as it should be.

Some of these terms may need explaining. Glucose simply means sugar in the blood. The BUN reading could indicate some kind of kidney disorder. A higher creatinine result could mean the kidneys were not adequately filtering this element from the blood. However, the GFR is considered the best method for both measuring kidney function and staging kidney disease.

The GFR is also important since the dosage of any medication you take may have to be adjusted for the level of kidney function revealed by the GFR. Many drugs exit your body via the kidneys. That means if your kidney function is reduced, these drugs are staying in your body longer than they need to since they are being eliminated more slowly, so you may need to take less of them or take the medication less often.

The percentage of kidney function is measured by comparing the amount of waste produced in your urine to the amount of waste found in your blood stream. To be perfectly clear, this test showed that my kidneys were functioning at a Stage 2 Kidney Disease Level. Panic time for me!

Sodium, potassium, chloride, phosphate, calcium, magnesium and carbon dioxide are all electrolytes that the kidneys help keep in balance and, according to this blood test, were. The anion gap deals with the body's acidity. A high reading for the anion gap could indicate renal failure. At this point, I decided the rest of the Comprehensive Metabolic Panel was just too technical for me. But the not knowing was worse than the knowing, so I forced myself to investigate.

Protein, Total looks for an indication of kidney or liver function. I was so glad I took the time to research this. **Albumin**, produced in the liver, deals with a certain pressure between blood and tissue fluids. Globulin was being tested for any degenerative, inflammatory and infectious processes. Ah, CKD is a degenerative disease.

I was beginning to feel I was re-inventing the wheel, but knew I was still a little too fragile to understand what the doctor was explaining, even if I did take notes. So, I kept on researching. It turned out that a low reading for the Albumin/Globulin Ratio [ALB/GLOB RATIO] could indicate a liver problem. Notice you're not being tested solely for CKD problems, but also for anything that might exacerbate your CKD condition.

Calcium does more for our bodies than just keeping our bones healthy and growing as we were told when we were children. Calcium also deals with muscle contraction, trauma, infection and stress. Too much calcium in CKD patients can lead to a certain bone disease and/or heart disease.

The following tests have quick explanations:

❖ Alkaline phosphatase is a protein found in the body's tissues. If it is elevated, a liver, bone or intestinal problem, possibly cancer, is indicated.

❖ Alt and Ast are tests to indicate liver damage or dysfunction by detecting the presence of these enzymes in your circulation when they should have remained in the liver.

❖ Bilirubin, Total is the test to see just how much bilirubin from damaged or old, dead red cells remained in the blood when the hemoglobin broke down. A higher than normal reading for this test could mean a chemical imbalance which would need to be addressed.

Tsh w/reflex to Free T4 Tsh

I am not kidding: when I first read the name of this test, I thought of a protest sign demanding freedom for some kind of revolutionary who had been jailed despite popular support. I was getting tired of trying to understand what I didn't understand and cracking silent jokes to relieve the tension. What this test is really for is to see if the T3 test comes back abnormal. If it does, the lab needs to run another thyroid test. That test, the T4, is a further thyroid test which looks for specific causes of the abnormality.

Urogram w/Rflx Micro and Culture

Normal urine has a color - pale to dark yellow or amber - and is clear. That much I readily understood. I giggled when I read "specific gravity" since I was reading quickly and saw that as specific gravy. The giggling only confirmed that I was becoming even tenser with all this new information, but I felt I needed to know what the tests were. The Urogram w/Rflx Micro and Culture is a serious test for kidney patients: a specific gravity above the reference range may mean renal impairment.

The only thing I really wanted to know about in this section was the word "Moderate" with the P.A.'s question mark over it. It turns out that leukocyte esterase simply means that there are white blood cells in the urine. White blood cells fight infection. I had a plain, old, garden variety infection that a dose of **antibiotic** would take care of. It didn't indicate anything serious or associated with the kidneys.

I decided I'd better understand the other tests, too:

❖ A positive nitrite reading might mean bacteria.
❖ The Ph, Urine tests are to check for urinary tract infections or to see if you're at risk for **kidney stones**. Despite the in range result, I ended up with a teeny, little kidney stone that summer.
❖ Blood, Protein, and Glucose are Urine, Qual. tests. None of these three substances is usually found in the urine, although **glucose** may appear in very

minute quantities. All could indicate kidney disease if found in the urine.

I thought I remembered what ketones were but checked anyway. I was right that their presence may indicate diabetes, but I did not know they could also indicate starvation. Urobilinogen and bile deal with liver disease. I realized this new physician was taking very good care of me. There were numerous tests to examine the liver function, and she had picked up the low estimated GFR.

Urinalysis, Microscopic

I already knew about white blood cells and red ones from the CBC, but I didn't recognize epithelial. An increased number of these cells in the urine may indicate a kidney problem. There seemed to be so many possible, but not necessary definite, indicators of kidney disease in all these tests.

Bacteria were things I was familiar with, but Hyaline Casts were not. Apparently, these are normally in your urine, but a larger number of them may - here's that word again - possibly be an indication of kidney disease. The casts themselves are small tubules or very, very small tubes.

I didn't know what to do with all this information, all these may indicates. I was researched out and had a tenuous hold on only one or two of what these tests meant in terms of kidney disease, although I understood the liver tests more clearly. It was peculiar that I'd never bothered to find out more about them before. They somehow didn't seem all that important until now when I might have CKD. I needed my doctor and my notebook. I made another appointment, so she could explain again what these tests meant and I could take notes while she did.

CHAPTER 3:

The Doctor's Appointment That Led to a Nephrologist

Let me think! The doctor is talking about kidney disease and the triglyceride test result is out of range. I was given a pamphlet on triglycerides and told to lower that number within the next month. This was getting so complicated. I thought we were looking for kidney disease. The booklet told me that triglyceride was a bad fat, just like LDL cholesterol, which could affect my heart and blood vessel health, and that cardiovascular disease [read heart and arteries] is the number one killer of Americans. Great, now it's not only the liver and the kidneys I need to worry about, but also the heart and arteries. I mean my liver, kidneys, heart and arteries.

It was made clear that lifestyle changes just might do the trick as far as the triglyceride number. Other than a little dancing here and there, I no longer did much exercising by now. Okay, I resolved, I would again dance vigorously several times a week. My doctor agreed, but gently suggested I add some kind of movement every day. I had unwittingly become a sedentary person – a couch potato. What could I do? I'd figure it out later. I was not to smoke, drink, or do drugs. That wasn't going to make any difference because I didn't do any of that anyway.

Dietary changes were necessary, too. I was to eat at least five servings of fruit and vegetables daily [You'll see later that this is not in accordance with the renal diet]. Grain products such as whole wheat bread and brown rice were to be added right away. I had no argument with that. My grandfather had been a miller in the Ukraine, so my love of bread must have been in the genes. There were other restrictions that didn't seem to be problematic until I received the renal diet a short time later. Many of the restricted foods on that diet were suggested to help control the triglyceride number.

My head was spinning. I'd thought it was enough to eat fresh, organic food and rarely ate meat because it just didn't taste that good to me.

Body Mass Index [BMI] which involved all those numbers - the nemesis of my life – was now going to be a daily part of my life. The BMI formula was something about your weight divided by the sum of your height in inches squared times 703. I think. I have researched and researched this, but still do not understand it. I did discover later on that there are free BMI Calculators online, such as the one on the United States Department of Health and Human Services' website [http://www.nhlbisupport.com/bmi/bminojs.htm], so you really only need to know your height and weight. If I'd known that at the time, I just might not have felt so overwhelmed.

I may have neglected to mention that according to my BMI at this time, I was obese. I don't know which was more of a shock – that I had such serious medical issues, or that I was obese.

Come to think of it, it's a good thing at this point that I didn't know about the weighing and measuring of your food that is involved with the renal diet. There's not only the counting of food groups, but the number of servings for each group and then the calorie count. I was already swimming in that foreign sea of numbers with just my blood and urine test results.

Trans-fatty acids would have to go, too. I readily agreed thinking it might be nice to know what I just agreed to. The doctor took a look at my eyes wandering around the office and realized I had no clue. She explained, with help from the pamphlet she'd handed to me about lowering your triglycerides, that trans-fatty acids are found in fast foods. Damn! No more McDonald's drive through breakfasts when I was running late to get to work, no more cookies and doughnuts which I naively thought wouldn't be a problem to cut out, no more fried food like the calamari I liked to share with one daughter or the onion rings I liked to share with my other daughter. It's a good thing that I started cutting these foods out right away because it made adhering to the renal diet a little bit easier later on.

Between the food and exercise changes, I was able to lower the triglyceride number to within the acceptable range in just a month. Unfortunately, at the same re-test my GFR was even lower and my BUN higher – not good - yet my creatinine was within range. It was time for a nephrologist. I also noticed I'd lost a pound. Was I that worried? It doesn't sound like a lot, but I'd been the same exact obese weight for over two years.

Being the thorough doctor that she was, my primary care physician also sent me for an **ultrasound** to take a look at what was going on inside. This uncovered a mild fatty infiltration of the liver. Was I in trouble here, too? It wasn't as bad as it sounded. It seemed a mild fatty infiltration of the liver was fairly common, occurring in almost 20% of the population and could be helped by losing weight. Obesity is one of the most usual causes of this condition. The obesity handwriting was on the wall for me.

That one pound loss also seemed to have had a slight benefit on my BMI. It was enough to convince me I should really work on the weight. Remember, I was still grasping at straws here. I kept an eye on this in my doctor visit reports and saw right there – in black and white – that as my weight went down, so did the BMI and the blood pressure.

I began requesting copies of my doctor visit reports as well as my blood and urine tests so I could have my own file at home and stay on top of whatever I needed to. With these copies, my home files would be much more thorough. I was feeling burned by my previous P.A.'s failure to pick up on the low readings for the estimated GFR and felt I had to be my own case manager. I still do and find both the nephrologist and my primary care physician agree with me.

Not a single doctor that I've seen for a test or a consultation has ever refused or been difficult about making certain I receive these copies. Most have encouraged me to keep my own, thorough medical files at home. I suspect it may have made life easier for these doctors, too, since there was no calling other doctors to fax reports or requesting them from labs. I had them and could fax them over to whichever doctor needed to see them immediately.

Since they are so highly personal, I decided not to include a Patient Exam from my own files but to describe one instead. My doctor visit reports, or Patient Exam reports, are usually several pages long and on my doctor's letterhead. They are factual accounts of you as a patient and are fairly cut and dry. The words I capitalized here are those that are capitalized on a Patient Exam.

They start with the date and then my current status: name; date of birth [DOB]; age; medications and dosages [including supplements and over the counter medications]; allergies; vitals - height, weight, BMI, temperature, pulse, blood pressure; smoker or not; and chief complaint or why I was seeing the doctor for this appointment.

The Patient Exam also included whether or not I had an Advanced Directive, a durable power of attorney for healthcare decisions or a health care proxy. In other words, you give someone else the power to make health care decisions for you if you can't, and, if so, what kind.

The History section was broken down into Pertinent Past Medical History; Surgical History; Family History; Social History including alcohol, caffeine, tobacco and drug use; Number of Children, Martial Status, Sexual History; Education and Employment; and the number of times a week I Exercise. Again, just facts.

Patient Exam reports are also called notes or doctor's visits reports. Make certain you check them for accuracy. For example, I've never taught high school in my new home state, but these reports had me doing so for five years. While it was just a simple transcription error, it completely obliterated my contact with asbestos that doctors know NYC school teachers were exposed to. My doctors, especially the nephrologist, should know about my exposure to this friable substance since it just might impact my disease. While this may not be considered a factor in developing CKD now, future research may change what we now consider the facts.

The second page of the Patient Exam is usually where the visit information begins. The first part of that is called the HPI, which means History of Present Illness. It included who I was as far my age, sex, and present medical state, why I made this appointment and my present medical conditions and medications. This section may include previous treatment for these problems, and what I planned to do as far as future treatment for them. Again, check for both accuracy and completeness. At one point, I found a disease listed here I could not pronounce, much less define. As it turned out, this disease did not exist. It was just a typographical error.

Then came the Review of Systems [ROS]. My primary care physician asked me questions about my constitution, the functional habits of my body such as weight changes, fever or chills. The cardiac part of my health was covered with questions about chest pain or palpitations. Finally, the lungs were referred to with questions about coughs, shortness of breath and **dyspnea**.

On my initial visit, the ROS was more inclusive with questions about my eyes, ears, nose, throat, and the following systems: respiratory, gastrointestinal, **genitourinary**, musculoskeletal, **integumentary**, neurological, psychiatric and endocrine. That made sense because this doctor had never met me before and needed to make her own assessment rather than trust that of my previous doctor.

It's very much like going to a new auto mechanic. He or she may ask for your car's history, but then the mechanic would want to personally examine the car. While there are car faxes about a car's history, there isn't a body fax about your body's history yet. Ah, where is Bones ("Star Trek") when you need him?

The next section, The Report of the Physical Examination, was based on the doctor's observations and palpitations of my body. It included a general appraisal of my appearance, and specifics about my neck, heart, lungs, abdomen and extremities. This is the poking around part of your visit. Again, it was more comprehensive on my initial visit and included the eyes, respiratory and lymphatic systems, skin, neurological and psychiatric aspects of my health.

The report continued with whatever Diagnostic Procedures had been done. On my first visit, this consisted of reviewing the charts from my previous physician, and the lab and abdominal ultrasound results. That was enough to jolt me, but more because I didn't yet know what any of this meant for me than that the actual results were devastating. I hadn't taken any of this information into account before.

The Assessments following this section intrigued me because they all began with numbers which I later discovered to be diagnosing codes. At this point, they were more of the mystery my health presented to me. I was lost in more numbers. After examining these numbers for a while, I realized the terms next to them identified the codes. I recognized hypertension and right shoulder pain, but should I be as worried as I was by hyperlipidemia (I needed to get home and research this.), renal insufficiency, and fatty liver? This last one was somehow offensive as if my obesity were being rubbed in my face.

I looked at The Plan. What? Now I might have rotor cuff disease, too? Apparently, that was how my family doctor interpreted the pain in my right shoulder. Why couldn't I just have a sore shoulder? How did the suspicion of one disease lead to the suspicion of all these others? I was to see my old friend, the orthopedic surgeon, about this.

I was able to figure out from the plan that hyperlipidemia was high cholesterol. I was already taking Lovastatin to control my high cholesterol so it was just going to be retested in three months.

Then I saw it - "Referred her to Nephrology for consultation treatment." I was going to see a nephrologist, a doctor who specialized in kidney diseases and HBP. I had both. My senses started tingling. I was sure this meant death (I just didn't realize it meant eventual death, the same kind every living creature faces). I was sure this meant immediate dialysis, but I didn't know exactly what dialysis meant. I just knew I had a colleague who had gone to a dialysis center several times a week and died anyway. I had to stop this spiraling hysteria right now, or I'd paralyze myself with this out of control fear. I had to educate myself about this nephrology stuff.

I barely noticed that the fatty liver might be remedied by a low fat diet. I was too busy obsessing about renal insufficiency. Later, in the Follow Up and Labs section, I noticed I was to have a follow up in three months after another Comprehensive Metabolic Panel [CMP] and Lipid Panel and, of course, a visit to my friendly, neighborhood nephrologist. The referral for this specialist was here, too. It was also noted that no injections or prescriptions **[scripts]** were given at this visit.

I asked the very few questions I could formulate. My poor doctor wanted to help so much, but most of these questions dealt directly with renal disease, and she couldn't answer them. However, she somehow maintained an encouraging attitude which helped calm my internal furor enough to allow me to make the call, the one I dreaded, to the nephrologist for an appointment.

CHAPTER 4:

How to Further Frighten the
New CKD Patient

Being no fool (or so I thought at the time), I immediately contacted the American Association of Kidney Patients asking that they send me whatever pamphlets they had. And they did. And I started quaking in my boots again.

Being the wonderfully informative – even if I wasn't ready to accept or even understand the material – organization that they are, they sent me pamphlet after pamphlet: *Kidney Beginnings: A Patient's Guide to Living with Reduced Kidney Function, When Your Loved One is Depressed, Understanding Depression in Kidney Disease, Understanding Anemia in Kidney Disease,* and *Understanding High **Phosphorus** and Your Treatment Options.* I haven't even included the ones about dialysis or transplantation options.

Two pamphlets about depression? Did that mean I was bound to become depressed because I had CKD? I later learned that depression may be a part of the stress of becoming a CKD patient. Overnight, you become a special person with special needs. I asked so many questions of my nephrologist that he feared this was what was happening to me. It wasn't, but it seems it could have been.

As a CKD patient, you have to think about everything: how much of each kind of food, which foods at all, over the counter medications, exercises, sometimes even integrating rest periods into your day. You need to stay in balance which means you are constantly changing the dosage of vitamins, minerals and medications based on the latest results of your blood and urine tests. Maybe you need more **vitamin D** this quarter or less calcium. It's so individual. Sometimes, this depression can be caused by something as simple as not being able to admit you are overwhelmed and need help. You need to relearn that you are more than this disease.

The steps to accepting this diagnosis reminded me of people dealing with death. The first is shock. Yes, that was me. I was dumbfounded. Then, there's grief. I think I may have skipped this step by researching instead. After that, there is usually denial, but again I was so quick to research that I found myself not grieving but dreading what I thought was going to be imminent dialysis.

I remembered reading somewhere that denial does have a purpose as long as it is not never-ending. It helps you cope with this news until you can deal with it. Just be sure you don't use denial as a reason for non-compliance with your nephrologist's and nutritionalist's directions. It was the research that led me into acceptance. This was my life, and I would learn to adapt to it because I didn't like the alternative.

It took me about a year to pick up these pamphlets again after initially reading them. They do not go into that much depth, are obviously meant to be helpful, and are gentle introductions to the topics. But I wasn't ready. I put them away and ignored them until I decided to write this book. Then I looked at them a third time – and still felt the dread that this was going to be my future. For all the information available to me about my disease and all these educational booklets, I couldn't help thinking that depression and dialysis or transplantation was going to be my immediate future.

I was an optimist by nature, so why all the pessimism? I believed in learning everything I could about anything that affected my life, so why the rigid attempt to shut this out? I had a mental image of a large hand being held up in the universal STOP mode in front of this information. Maybe I needed a less official approach. After all, the American Association of Kidney Patients calls itself "The Voice of All Kidney Patients," and I had never been a joiner.

I'd been told about http://www.DaVita.com at my doctor's office. This was a website from a private company that provided both the much dreaded dialysis and the much needed kidney education. Maybe that wouldn't be so foreboding for me. I went to the website and clicked on every possible thing I could click on. This was a little better, but it was a dot com – a for profit site. Maybe it was one that offered all this information so that when you needed dialysis, you would turn to them since they had been so helpful all along.

And what, if anything, was wrong with that? I wasn't as upset by this site as I was by the American Association of Kidney Patients' [AAKP] material. AAKP included a magazine with recipes and another with current articles. I'd given them little thought once I'd been alarmed by the other pamphlets, but decided now that hadn't been fair.

A year and a half later, I revisited the site and found that I somehow managed to overlook their entire educational aspect. Yes, DaVita is a profit-making company, but they also aim to educate the CKD patient about the disease and how to stay as healthy as possible - not only during dialysis - but before. In other words, during the early CKD stages. They have recipes, explanations of the value of watching potassium or sodium intake and how to do so in your kitchen. There are videos, articles and links. Now that my initial fear had finally decreased, I'd suggest everyone who has CKD log on to http://www.davita.com, but only when you're ready.

I was apparently a lucky patient (How's that for a contradiction in terms?). I had the time to deny, then admit my fear, work through it and learn as much as I could about my condition. Of course, in the interim, my doctor explained more to me as did my nutritionist. I knew no one else with the information I sought and the internet was alternately my best friend and teacher or my worst enemy and nemesis, depending upon my state of mind on any particular day.

I was flagging under the dearth or glut of information depending on the day. I was having trouble tying all these bits of CKD information together. My nutritionist noticed I was down during an appointment and asked why. When I told her, she asked me to wait a moment and then ran out of the room only to return with more magic: a list of helpful websites that included http://ikidney.com – a renal support network - and, more importantly to me, http://www.kidneyschool.org. That was something I could relate to. I was a teacher. I was comfortable with anything that had school in the title.

I eagerly pulled the site up on my computer and wasn't disappointed. It was a bit simplistic, but I needed that at this point while I was still dealing with my emotions. I'd both taught and taken online college courses and was comfortable with the format, not that you need this experience to make use of this website. I went back several times to make sure I understood what I'd just learned.

I could do this at my own rate. If I had a writing deadline (I am also a writer) and couldn't work on kidney school that day, it would be waiting right there on my computer for me the next day. If I was having an emotionally overwhelmed day, I could skip it until the mood passed. But it was there, and it explained. If you're computer literate or can get someone to work the computer for you, I'd strongly urge you take a look.

Gradually, very gradually, as I began to understand more and more about my disease in the privacy of my own home and at my own rate, I got stronger emotionally and was able to look at more complicated or technical sites. I began to read novels that had characters with CKD. It wasn't an easy task to find them, but the card catalogue – which is usually electronic – and the librarian were great helps until I figured out how to find them myself via an ever narrowing subject search.

I continued to look for books like this one (using the search terms *medical self-help* or *medical narrative*, just in case you were wondering), but I didn't find them. I began to think my nephrologist was right. I'd have to write one. But I wanted to make sure I understood the information before I started writing and so researched even more.

I thought www.kidney.org would be helpful since it is the official website of the National Kidney Foundation, but it was a little too social for me. I was one of those people who would rather not be a member of any group if I could help it. I was drawn to some of the educational parts of the site, which I found after clicking on patients, then Chronic Kidney Disease.

The American Kidney Fund at www.kidneyfund.org, while a helpful site, also wasn't my cup of tea. I shied away from the obvious request for donations even as I realized they'd need money to continue their work. Was it the ads? The busy website? I knew it was a valuable site but not for me. I'd urge you to visit as many different CKD sites as you can. You'll find some – although sometimes even one is enough – that resonate with you.

I was down to the last website on the list the nutritionist had given me: Kidney and Urological Diseases at the United States Department of Health and Human Services. The officious title itself was enough to make me leery, but I dutifully went to the URL: http://www2.niddk.nih.gov. I discovered that by clicking on Kidney & Urological Diseases on the homepage, I was sent to http:kidney.niddk.nih.gov which I could have typed in to avoid the homepage entirely. At this address, I found easily understood fact sheets, educational material, an awareness and prevention program, and was even directed to additional sources of information about CKD. It was also simple to navigate on this site.

I was pleased to see the variety of brochures available from the different sites. I wasn't so sure I really wanted to learn about dialysis and transplantation yet, but I could still learn about the hows and whys of CKD by requesting only the brochures I was comfortable reading. I was ready to learn more, and this helped pace my learning.

That decision also helped me decide not to discuss dialysis or transplantation in this book. There were numerous books, brochures, and websites that dealt with these weighty issues and besides, I wasn't there yet. What could I write about my experience with them if I had none?

That's also the reason I don't deal with children's CKD in this book. My children are fortunate enough not to have this disease and, I have to admit that I found it harder to deal with the thought of a child with this disease than my having it. Some might say I'm old, and have lived my life. I say I'm older, and have lived a great deal of my life, something a child has not yet had the time to do.

I did contact MedCure. This company will pick up your body after you die, harvest your tissues and organs for research and education and cremate the rest of you to give the ashes to whomever you designate. They will also scatter your ashes, if you'd prefer. This costs nothing, but they will test your body before accepting it. According to their website, they will be testing for "...infectious disease or condition such as Hepatitis B or C, HIV/AIDS, active tuberculosis, history of illegal drug use, incarceration or severely under or overweight at the time of death."

MedCure is the company I contacted. I'm sure there are others. Their contract is a legal document under the Uniform Anatomical Gift Act and their home state's Oregon Anatomical Gift Statutes. I noticed there is such an organization in my home state, but it doesn't seem to matter where you live. I will die eventually, CKD or no CKD, and feel my children should not be burdened with additional decisions on my behalf at that time. This is a personal decision, but I did want you to know such places exist.

CHAPTER 5:

What Flows Through You

On the following page, you'll find a sample lab order for blood and urine tests to be performed after a 24 hour urine collection. These tests are important because both your diagnosis and your staging are based on them. The personal, nephrologist and lab information has been either covered or blackened out for privacy purposes. When I first looked at this, all I saw was numbers, numbers, numbers, especially since the words didn't mean anything to me.

I asked the nurse what they meant, and she started to explain. But we were interrupted every few minutes by other nurses, doctors or patients. I realized this was not going to be a five minute conversation. "Thanks, anyway," I concluded the conversation. "I can look it up at home." She did a double take and asked if I were sure I wanted to do that. In my ignorance, I assured her it was fine. This was clearly another case of not understanding what was involved in looking it up.

The Top Section

If you look at the top of the, actually at the only information remaining at the top now that the identifying information has been deleted, you'll see the hand written note on the left, *Do this 2 wks. prior to Dec. appt.* That was to be my next six month appointment.

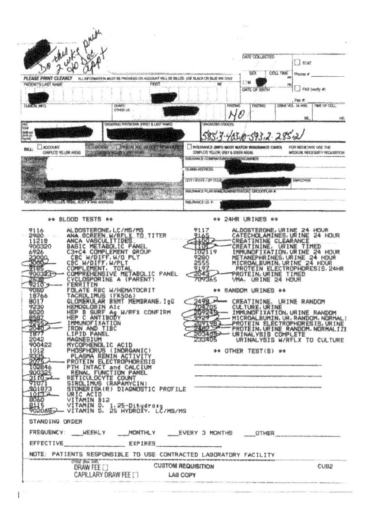

The two weeks mentioned seemed excessively early until a lab lost my specimens and the tests had to be repeated. I was lucky enough to receive a call from the nephrologist's office asking if I'd had the tests since they hadn't received the results, and I had an appointment in one week. With the explosion of CKD in the last decade, there's no guarantee that your doctor's office will have the time to offer this courtesy. Call to make certain that your lab results have been received a week or so before your appointment to prevent wasting your time and that of your doctor.

After many frustrating calls to the lab, their manager, their co-coordinator, and anyone else that might have been of help, it was determined that yes, indeed, the specimens – not the results, but the specimens – had been lost. I haven't been back to that particular very busy lab site since. While this is not a typical occurrence, you need to be vigilant that the very few times it may happen you can rectify the situation or repeat the tests in time for them to reach your nephrologist before your next appointment.

Another time, the specimens were located, but the results had been sent to the wrong doctor someone I'd never heard of who is probably still wondering why this new patient never made an appointment. I didn't go back to this lab site, either.

I've found a small satellite office of the same parent lab company that never seems to be all that busy which makes me feel the specimens and the results will be well looked after. This may not be true at all, but I like the psychological comfort it gives me.

Interesting tidbit: my first nephrologist felt I should be seen in the office once a year to discuss the test results after undergoing the tests, the second – and present – one felt six month visits would be a better option for me. Different doctors – different orders. Either way, the office visit would be to discuss what flowed through me.

Notice on the right side of the script, above the diagnosis codes, the word *No* written underneath *FASTING*. That was unlike my quarterly liver function blood test which was fasting and has since been changed to *Yes*, meaning nothing to eat or drink after midnight the day before your blood test. If you need lab tests for different doctors and for different purposes, read the script that you'll be bringing to the lab the day before so you know whether or not to fast.

In my case, my medications would not change the test results, so it was all right to take them the morning of the test. That's not true in all cases. Ask your doctor when you're given your script if fasting includes your **meds**.

I wanted to know exactly what my diagnoses codes meant. I wanted to understand the words associated with the numbers since I'm a word person, not a number person, so I used my computer. I discovered a site where these codes are explained. It's the site for the International Classification of Diseases, 10th Revision. You can identify each of your codes at http://apps.who.int/classifications/apps/icd/icd10online/.

Libraries also carry a copy of *The International Classification of Diseases, Clinical Modification : ICD-CM* [**ICD**] although it may be a reference book meaning it cannot be taken out of the library. The call number is 616.1612. But, then again, most libraries offer the free use of a computer for their members.

As you can see, I have a host of codes. Most kidney patients do since there are so many accompanying "gifts" from, or contributing to, the disease. The ICD is clearly, numerically organized. For example, my first code is: 585.3, so I followed these steps to find my diagnosis.

❖ When I went to the *ICD* online, I clicked on 580-629 and discovered this group of codes deals with Diseases of the Genitourinary System.

❖ Within that range of diagnoses, I clicked on 580-589 which revealed that these codes deal with Nephritis, Nephrotic Syndrome, and Nephrosis. Nephro means kidney.

❖ Refining the diagnosis code even more, I clicked on 585 which turned out to be Chronic Kidney Disease.
❖ From the menu under 585, I clicked .3 to discover that this is Stage 3 of the disease.

So I have Stage 3 Chronic Kidney Disease.

I researched my second diagnosis in exactly the same manner:

❖ 403.10 falls within the range of 390-459, **Circulatory Diseases**.
❖ 401-405 deal specifically with Hypertensive Disease.
❖ Narrowing the diagnosis down to 403 brings us to Hypertensive Kidney Disease.
❖ The .10 lands me at Benign Hypertensive Renal Disease without renal failure.

The drop down menus under each more generalized code made this a painless process.

By the time I got to the third diagnosis code, I couldn't think of anything else that might be wrong with me. My third diagnosis was 593.2.

❖ I dutifully clicked on 580-629, which I already knew from my first diagnosis code is the category for Diseases Of The Genitourinary System.
❖ On the dropdown menu, I clicked 590-599 which turned out to be Other Diseases Of Urinary System. Other Diseases of Urinary System? What was this?

❖ I clicked 593*. That was Other Disorders of Kidney and Ureter, which didn't help much. The asterisk referred me to the second volume of *The ICD* for the specific Medicare or **Medicaid** code [which surprised me since I do not use either as my insurance, but there seems to be no other code for this].

❖ Finally, the .2 told me this was a **Cyst** of Kidney Acquired. Oh, right. I vaguely remembered the nephrologist mentioning I had a cyst.

My last diagnosis code was 285.21. *The ICD* trail for that is:

❖ 280-289 - Diseases Of The Blood And Blood-Forming Organs (Oh no! I had a blood disease, too?)

❖ 285 - Other and Unspecified Anemias.

❖ 21* - Anemia in Chronic Kidney Disease. The asterisk means the same as it does for 593.2 above. After a sigh of relief that this wasn't worse, I realized that I had always been borderline anemic and the CKD exacerbated that.

This took a lot less time on the computer than it took to write about the process. It's just a matter of click, click, click. Of course, you may need a good medical dictionary [see Chapter 13] to understand your final diagnoses. While you may have the same diagnoses I do, you also may have other diagnoses that I don't. You research them the same way. The benefit of actually going to the library is that you have a reference librarian to help if you find yourself in research trouble.

The Blood Tests

You won't need to do much research to understand the lower part of the lab order since the numerical codes have their definitions right next to them. Again, all you need is a medical dictionary. Only the circled numbers are the tests performed under this script. Mine were:

3000 - CBC W/Diff, W/Plat. This is the same test as the one in my original blood tests.

900323 - Comprehensive Metabolic Panel. This is the same test that my primary care physician ordered and is discussed in Chapter 2, except for the more specific tests she hadn't ordered then.

9210 - Ferritin, which refers to the test of this protein that stores your iron until your body needs it. An infection can interfere with its function, so an abnormal reading doesn't necessarily mean there's a problem. Your doctor may ask you to take a regiment of antibiotics and then retest. This, I know from personal experience.

9225 - Immunofixation uses antibodies to identify the types of proteins or antibodies separated by protein electrophoresis. Your doctor needs the information garnered by test 2075 [Protein Electrophoresis explained later on this list] to make sense of this. It's fairly technical medically, but you can make use of a medical dictionary if you'd like more information about this particular test.

2040 - Iron and TIBC. Iron TIBC stands for Total Iron Binding Capacity. It shows if there is an abnormal amount of iron in the blood by measuring how well the protein transferrin is carrying iron in the blood. Iron is what is used in the bone marrow to produce red blood cells. Low iron contributes to anemia, a not unusual byproduct of CKD.

2075 - Protein Electrophoresis separates elements of your blood into individual components. Immunofixation identifies the proteins found in this test. That's how 9225 and 2075 work together: 2075 separates the individual components of your blood, while 9225 identifies the types of proteins or antibodies found there.

3110 - Reticulocyte Count measures how fast the bone marrow produces red blood cells [the reticulocytes, or immature red blood cells in the title of the test] and releases them into the blood. Again, a low red blood cell count contributes to anemia. Your doctor may need to order iron supplements or synthetic iron intravenously, if necessary. Unfortunately, extra iron may lead to constipation, so talk this over with your doctor should your results for this test suggest you need extra iron.

1013 - Uric Acid levels in the blood can indicate that you're at risk for gout, kidney stones, or kidney failure. It's the kidney's job to filter uric acid from the body. A buildup means the kidneys are not doing their job well. This doesn't seem to be foolproof since I hadn't had elevated uric acid levels in the blood but did experience a kidney stone.

902068 - Vitamin D, 25 Hydroxy, LC/MS/MS. I can't resist telling you I burst out laughing again – obviously, a much needed relief by this time - when I read this. I immediately visualized a Hydrox cookie being tested. In reality, the test is just what it says it is: a test of the vitamin D in your body, since calcium production is dependent on Vitamin D.

❖ The kidneys produce calcitrol which is the active form of vitamin D. The kidneys are the organs that transfer this vitamin from your food and skin [sunshine provides it to your skin] into something your body can use.

❖ Both vitamin D and calcium are needed for strong bones. It is yet another job of your kidneys to keep your bones strong and healthy.

❖ Should you have a deficit of Vitamin D, you'll need to be treated for this, in addition for any abnormal level of calcium or phosphates. The three work together.

❖ Vitamin D enables the calcium from the food you eat to be absorbed in the body. CKD may leech the calcium from your bones and body.

❖ Phosphate levels can rise since this is stored in the blood and the bones as is calcium. With CKD, it's hard to keep the phosphate levels normal, so you may develop itchiness since the concentration of urea builds up and begins to crystallize through the skin. This is called **pruritus**.

Those are the blood tests ordered for me. Some of yours may be different or the same. You can research yours the same way I did by simply entering the name of the test in your search bar and then choosing the site you want to look at. I chose the most comprehensive definitions so I could thoroughly understand the test before writing about it, but you may choose the easiest to understand. There's no sense having an authoritative definition if you haven't a clue what it means.

Somewhere along the line, one of your doctors may order an A1C test. This measures how well your blood sugar has been regulated for the two or three months before the test. That's possible because the glucose adheres to the red blood cells. This is important since quite a few CKD patients develop the disease from diabetes.

The 24 Hour Urine Collection Tests

There's also a 24 hour urine collection analysis requested on this script. Surprisingly, the written instructions you are given about how to collect the urine may not be clear. If so, ask. It's better to take a few extra minutes of the P.A. or **M.A.**'s time for an explanation than having to collect the urine all over again due to contamination. Your nephrologist will have already given you the container for collection and, if you are female, a collection seat (for lack of a better term). This is something you place over your open toilet seat to insure you don't waste any of the urine.

Well, that is, after the first urination of the day. That one goes directly down the toilet and is not part of the collection. You'll also be instructed to do what should be obvious: wash your hands both before and after you urinate and be sure not to allow any foreign substance like menstrual blood, toilet paper, or fecal matter to get into your urine collection.

You'll need to refrigerate the specimens as you collect them during the 24 hour urine collection. It's important to catch all the urine you produce during this time period [except for the first urination on the first day] since the amount, or volume, of urine you produce is used in the equation that determines your stage of CKD.

On a personal note, you've got to make certain the lab understands your doctor's orders and your doctor had really ordered the tests you're taking. I recently had the unhappy experience of having my 24 hour urine collection tossed by the lab. It wasn't on the script I brought them from my nephrologist, and when they called his office at my insistence, they were told it wasn't time for that and not to accept it. At my next doctor's appointment when I told him what had happened, he said nothing - just pantomimed banging his head against the wall.

More tests that were ordered were:

1100 Creatinine Clearance - When compared to the amount of creatinine in your blood, this is the most accurate test to assess how well the kidneys are filtering the creatinine from your blood.

> ❖ Remember, creatinine is the waste product from muscle metabolism. The less creatinine in your urine, the more in your blood, which means the kidneys are not working as well as they should.

❖ You need to be aware that creatinine clearance values go down as you age. One source suggested 6.5 mL/min for every 10 years past age 20. You'll see your mL/min on your test results. The decrease in clearance values as you age meant quite a bit of figuring for me since I'm in my mid sixties. It only reaffirmed that you just can't get away from math with this disease.

1101- another creatinine test, but slightly different since the urine is timed. Because creatinine is not recycled in the blood, it is produced at a constant rate and only the kidneys filter it from the blood. This test is a more exact determination of how well or poorly the kidneys are functioning.

2043, Protein, Urine Timed - tests for protein in the urine during a specific time period, 24 hours in this case. Since one of the jobs of the kidneys is to filter the protein from your blood and then reabsorb it, there should be very little to no protein in your urine if your kidneys are functioning well.

The Random Urine Tests

Finally, there are the random urines. Think, "Pee in the cup." You'll be asked to do this, as well as give blood, when you bring your 24 hour urine collection to your lab. Oddly enough, in this case random refers to a special time of the day, namely the time of day you're producing a urine sample. While these are not as accurate as the 24 hour urine collection tests, they do allow your doctor to see how much of each element is being secreted when you urinate.

To illustrate the importance of this test, one summer I'd suffered infection after infection for a total of five. This necessitated quite a few random urine tests to watch the white blood count. When that count was elevated, an infection was present. When it wasn't, the antibiotics had accomplished their task and I was finally infection free.

2498 - deals with the creatinine that is voided in the urine at one specific time. In other words, this test measures the creatinine in one urine sample rather than during the entire 24 hour collection period.

209245 Immunofixation, Urine, Random - used to assess the state of your immune system. [Notice this was also tested in the blood.]

9929 Microalbumin, Ur, Random, Normal - tests for micro, or very small amounts, of albumin in the urine. Ur stands for urine. Albumin is a form of protein that is water soluble. Urine is a liquid, a form of water, so the albumin should have been dissolved. Protein in the urine may be an indication of kidney disease.

209198 Protein, Electrophoresis, Urine - serves the same purpose as the blood test for this. It separates the different components of protein in your urine, rather than in the blood.

209245 Immunofixation, Urine, Random - identifies the proteins found in the test explained above [209198 Protein, Electrophoresis, Urine].

2482 Protein, Urine Random, Normalized - similar to 2043 [Protein, Urine Timed]. The difference is that this measures the protein in one sample of your urine, rather than the entire 24 hour collection period's urine.

203405 Urinalysis, Complete - can't be part of the 24 hour collection due to the additives used to preserve the specimen. It is complete in another way. The urine is visually examined for color, transparency and odor. This is what you usually hear about as the urine test for drugs, but this also may catch signs of different diseases.

❖ Food and drugs can change the color of urine, but so can concentration or dilution of the urine. CKD patients are instructed to drink 64 ounces of liquid a day. Too much will make the color of your urine very light. Not enough will cause your urine to become a deep yellow.

❖ Cloudiness, rather than transparency, could mean kidney stones or the beginning of a phosphate or urate which may indicate a problem. Urate is a salt of the uric acid whose presence could indicate gout. The presence of either element could also mean that the sample has been un-refrigerated for too long or that a bacterial growth is present. Either way, it's an indication that more testing is needed.

❖ While unusual urine odor could be due to a plain, old, ordinary urinary tract infection, it might also be caused by ketone bodies in the urine. When the kidneys or liver break down fatty acids for energy, these are the by products which are used by the heart and brain for energy. There could be any number of causes for their presence, but the important part is that diabetes may be one of them.

Just a little bit more of this. The second part of the Complete Urinalysis deals with specific gravity of the urine which has been tested since abnormally diluted urine may indicate kidney disease. High specific gravity may indicate diabetes, which is one of the primary causes of CKD. My reaction to this was a big question mark about just what gravity was in the first place. It turned out to be the concentration of particles in the urine. Evaluating this helps evaluate your body's water balance and urine concentration.

The biochemical part of the urinalysis tests leukocytes, nitrates, Ph, proteins, ketones, urobilinogen, glucose, bilirubin, blood, and hemoglobin. To be as succinct as possible:

Leukocytes are one of the white blood cells that fight bacterial infection.

Nitrates present in the urine indicate bacteria and possibly diabetes.

High Ph may point to an over consumption of protein (I'm limited to five ounces a day) or CKD while low Ph may point to diabetes or dehydration.

Protein in the urine, or **proteinuria**, is one of the signs of kidney disease.

Ketone presence might be caused by uncontrolled diabetes.

High urobilinogen levels could be an indication of anemia.

High glucose levels might be the result of diabetes.

Bilirubin in the urine could be the result of liver failure.

Blood in the urine may indicate some kind of kidney disorder.

Hemoglobin in the blood may be a result of the breakdown of red cells. Hemoglobin in the red blood cells is what carries the oxygen through your body.

These are not the only causes for finding these elements in the urine. Should you decide you'd like to know more, try one of the online medical dictionaries among the websites listed in Chapter 13.

The final part of the urinalysis is microscopy and sediment. The sediment part refers to the particles that settle to the bottom when urine is allowed to stand for several hours and then examined under a microscope.

Albumin, stagnant urine, cellular debris and low urine filtration rate can cause a protein cast in the urinary sediment. Proteinuria can indicate kidney disease – as you probably remembered.

Urinary sediment doesn't usually contain crystals unless alkalization is present. As mentioned before, high Ph - or alkalization - may indicate kidney disease. But, then again, it may indicate not enough water intake or high water elimination.

There should be no micro-organisms in the urine sediment, but their presence may indicate a urinary tract infection – which is bacteria based - or kidney infection – which is yeast based. Other micro-organisms that may be detected are parasites, spermatozoa and mucus.

Now that the explanations of the tests are complete, you're probably aware of how many times I wrote *may indicate* and *can cause*. Understanding your blood and urine results is a more precise science than can be explained with a boiler plate list of what causes which problem or what each test may mean. Your doctor will be able to understand how the results of one test – or even one part of one test – implicate the other tests. The tests produce the pieces of your evaluation.

It's almost like a thousand piece jigsaw puzzle; some people are good at putting those together, others aren't. Your doctor is the one who's good at it, although it doesn't hurt to have a passing knowledge of just what is happening in what flows through your body.

CHAPTER 6:

The Nephrologist's Report

After an appointment with the nephrologist, he sent a report to my primary care physician and a copy of that report to me. Just as with the primary care physician's report, it was on letterhead stationary and began with all the identifying information: Patient Name, Date of Birth [DOB], Date of Service [DOS], Physician, and then my primary care doctor's name and address. Nothing earth shattering here, but this information does insure you're reading your own appointment report, and just as with the Patient Exam report from my family physician, there's too much personal information for me to include a sample in the book.

Following the identifying information is the History of Present Illness. This is important because this is your specialist writing about his specialty as it concerns your body. Since my body was no longer telling me what was going on inside it, someone had to, and I trusted my nephrologist. I've copied parts of it here, so I can explain it to you but deleted the personal information.

As you know, Gail is a [age omitted here] female who was initially seen by my partner [name omitted here] for management of Chronic Kidney Disease Stage 2, which is presumably secondary to **hypertensive nephrosclerosis.** She did a 24-hour urine collection on [date omitted here] showing **creatinine clearance** of 68.0 milliliters per minute [mL/min] with no significant proteinuria. During the interim her blood pressure seems to be controlled and here in the office it is at 110/62 [first number is the pressure of the blood during heartbeats, the second at rest between heartbeats]. She reported to me that she had **nephrolithiasis** per ultrasound but **asymptomatic**.

That was me in a nutshell as far as this doctor was concerned, and I thanked him for it. He reported my condition accurately, and I felt he was going to do his very best to help me slow this damned disease as much as possible.

Logically, the Past Medical History followed the History of Present Illness. These are the items concerning my CKD that my doctor included:

1. Chronic Kidney Disease Stage 2; estimated glomerular filtration rate of 60-65 mL/min presumably secondary to hypertensive nephrosclerosis.
2. Hypertension for more than 20 years.
3. **Dyslipidemia/ hypertriglyceridemia**.

This did not look so good for me. I was thrilled that the stage of my CKD was now 2 instead of 3 when I first read the notes because I thought I'd somehow managed to reverse the direction of my illness. My nephrologist burst my bubble by explaining that the stages changed due to the changes in the formula once I lost weight [weight is part of the formula as you'll see in Chapter 7]. The combination of CKD, HBP and high cholesterol placed me in the position of being a prime candidate for a heart attack or stroke. Me? Healthy me? Oh, right, that wasn't who I was anymore. This was truly a case of the truth hurts.

This brings me to some fairly lightweight information. I realize it's necessary to present a full medical picture of the patient but so little of it had to do with CKD. This information was included in: Past Surgical History, none of which relates to CKD, so I won't duplicate it here; Social History, which is similar to the one in my primary care doctor's report except that this one included my marital status, the medical history of my two grown daughters [I can only guess that this is requested to see if you are a carrier, since neither the internet nor the physicians I questioned could give me a satisfactory answer when I asked why this was included], and my former career; Family History which states the ages and causes of death for my parents, and ends with the following sentence: "There is no Chronic Kidney Disease or dialysis dependency in the family." Somehow, I didn't count myself lucky for being the first here.

The Review of Systems is very different from the one my family doctor wrote:

> Energy level and appetite are fair. No fever chills or night sweats. No acute visual disturbance or **oral thrush**. No chest pain at rest or exertion. No **paroxysmal nocturnal dyspnea**. No shortness of breath, chronic cough or **hemoptysis**. No **nausea**, vomiting, diarrhea or **melena**. No gross **hematuria** or **dysuria**. No foaminess in the urine. No difficulty with urine stream or sensation of incomplete bladder emptying. No lower extremity **edema** or **claudification**. No rash or unusual discoloration. No **effusion** or stiffness. No flank pain on urination [may be an indication of possible kidney trouble] or severe back pain. No severe headaches or **orthostatis**.

I realized immediately that, although I didn't understand all of this, it all dealt with the kidney problems or indications of kidney problems. It seems silly now, but that's when I realized that this doctor was, indeed, a specialist who treated serious disease and that this was real, I did have this serious disease. It was all so focused, so pointed in one direction. I think that's when I started to understand that I really needed to read a book that would help me grasp how this was happening to me, a book that neither my nephrologist, my librarian, nor I could find.

A list of allergies that didn't relate to CKD followed this mind changing information. Perfectly ordinary allergies that anyone could have. It seemed absurd they were even on the same page with the preceding information.

Below that, the nephrologist listed Current Medications. The only thing of note here is that I take Lovastatin 20 mg. **po** and **tid** for high cholesterol and Quinaretic 12.5/20 one tablet po and **bid** for HBP. These two disorders added to the CKD made my health picture pretty bleak, and I couldn't pretend it didn't anymore.

Patient Vitals are the next item in the report and include blood pressure, pulse and weight (can't get away from that in medical issues). They actually looked pretty good: well within range and appropriate (except for the weight, of course). So how could I have CKD? I kept coming back to that same thought. Now that I look at it in retrospect, I must have been a tough nut to crack: perfectly compliant, but alienated from the disease.

This is the complete entry for Physical Examination: General. Although a great deal of it is redundant, there is some new information that I'll explain.

> GENERAL: Appears as stated age. (I was insulted and decided that my youngish nephrologist just didn't appreciate older women who didn't look

their age.) Well nourished. (I was on a roll here
and decided he meant I was fat. This is actually
a referral to general wellness.)

HEENT [Head, Eyes, Ear, Nose, Throat]: No oral
thrush or ulcers. **Anicteric sclera.** Pink **conjunctiva**.

NECK: No **lymphadenopathy**. No **acanthosis
nigricans**.

CARDIOVASCULAR: Regular rate and rhythm, S1,
S2. No murmurs or rubs. No S3 or S4 **gallop**.

PULMONARY: Lungs are clear to **auscultation**
bilaterally. No wheezing, **rales** or **rhonchi**.

ABDOMEN: **Nondistended**. Soft.

EXTREMITIES: No lower extremity edema.
Acyanosis.

VASCULAR: Good **bounding** radial pulses, equal
and bilateral.

MUSCULOSKELETAL: No flank pain on palpa-
tion to the kidney. No paraspinal tenderness.

JOINTS: No effusion or stiffness of the hands.

SKIN: No rash or unusual discoloration.

NERUO: Able to stand without evidence of orthostatis. Steady gait.

PSYCH: Alert and oriented. Good insight.

There is nothing in the General Physical Examination that indicates I have CKD, but I do. Just as there is nothing in the Review of Systems that indicates I have CKD, but I do.

The LABORATORY DATA section of the doctor's report told a different story. It started with the date of my latest 24 hour urine creatinine clearance followed by a repeat of the readings.

The only ones that caught my eye were the BUN and creatinine. BUN means Blood Urea Nitrogen and may indicate a lowering of kidney function. While my reading of 20 was not the outside limit for someone in her 60s, it was close enough to the 23 that was the outside limit to make me nervous. As for creatinine, the more in your blood, the less the kidneys are filtering via your urine. 1.2 was out of range completely.

I already knew there was a problem, and I was doing my best to understand what it meant. My physician was a peculiar mix of cautionary and reassuring, but I couldn't seem to get my mind around this information and what it did and did not mean to me.

The next report was IMAGING STUDIES, in this case, an ultrasound. In addition to what was noted in my chart, an ultrasound is also used to determine the number of kidneys you have as well as any blockage, stones or abnormalities. It noted the size and appearance of my kidneys, then described the location and size of several benign cysts.

Now I had cysts on top of kidney disease? I was afraid to ask any questions for fear of more bad news except this turned out not to be such bad news. According to the nephrologist, cysts this small were of no consequence and ordinary. I've never felt more grateful to have some part of my body described as ordinary.

This was followed by the nephrologist's IMPRESSIONS, which started out with "Chronic Kidney Disease Stage 2, estimated glomerular filtration rate of 60-5 mL/min, likely secondary to presumed hypertensive nephrosclerosis." That means kidney damage due to HBP. (Even though it had been treated for the last 20 years? I did ask and was told simply, "Yes.").

Ironically, the next item in IMPRESSIONS was "Hypertension, well controlled on current medications." (I asked my question again and was told "yes" again.) Then there was mention of the cysts. Surprisingly, I also had iron deficiency without anemia. I somehow never connected my **fatigue** with kidney disease, but I was learning. My history of Dyslipidemia and my nephrolithiasis were mentioned, too.

Finally, the nephrologist's RECOMMENDATIONS. These included starting ferrous sulfate [iron] 325 mg. po at noon. Why noon? It seems you're meant to take this with a meal to minimize the chance of stomach upset. I suppose that made sense, but I was alternately teaching and acting at night, so noon was not a meal time for me. I went to sleep later and woke up later, so had lunch later with this night work schedule.

The vitamin C I had been taking was eliminated since it has high **oxalate** consistency which could cause further **nephrolithiasis**.

I had read of Omega 3 therapy being helpful in retarding the development of CKD and discussed this with my doctor. In this section of the nephrologist's report, he agreed that I could safely take 1200 mg. one tablet po bid

Here's a tricky one: I was to continue drinking at least 64 ounces of fluid [eight cups] a day but not more. Yes, I did start keeping track. I knew a cup of coffee was eight ounces, and I had two a day. That left me with 48 ounces which I kept to water unless I had four ounces of soy milk with my morning cereal. This is covered in more depth in Chapter 8: **The Renal Diet**.

The report, of course, ended with a one – two punch: I would need to exercise for at least 30 minutes a day and possibly decrease food portions, so I could lose weight (all right already! I got it!) for better blood pressure and renal function. Below that were my provider's name and other information identifying the electronic file.

Although I had carefully looked up every term I didn't know and had sat with this report for days while I did, I felt like I'd been run over by a truck – a big one. That's when I decided (yet again) I had to research everything I could about this disease. I read, I Googled, I sat in the library right next to the reference librarian, and I made a pest of myself at my doctor's office via phone calls and unscheduled visits – not the way to endear yourself to someone you need on your side.

In an unusual way, this paid off. I discovered I couldn't find what I wanted in one book, and it took too long to extract one bit of information from this book and another from that. I didn't see the purpose of every newly diagnosed CKD patient hoeing the same row. I decided to take my doctor's challenge: I would write that book I needed about Early Stage CKD.

CHAPTER 7:

The Estimated GRF

The symptoms of kidney disease don't show up until you've lost most of your kidney function. That's when you'll experience the fatigue that's not always a result of anemia, the muscle cramps that usually - but not always - present themselves in your calves, nausea, vomiting, appetite loss, easy bruising, itching and the shortness of breath when you exert yourself. If you're like me, you started feeling them as soon as you read about them, but they weren't really there. It was a classic case of medical student syndrome. That's when you are convinced you have the disease (or, in my case, the symptoms) as soon as you learn about it. Actually, according to my nephrologist, I'm probably at least 20 years away from such symptoms. So how do the doctors know I have CKD?

It's all in the numbers, the numbers of your estimated GRF that is. But what is the GRF, and why is it estimated? Isn't medicine an exact science? It seems not.

GRF means the Glomerular Filtration Rate. Big help, isn't it? Filtration Rate sounds easy enough, but what is a Glomerular? The dictionary tells us that filtrate is the part of a liquid that passed through a filter. So, glomerular filtration measures the filtrate from the glomerular.

According to *The Gale Encyclopedia of Medicine*, a glomerular is a small tuft of blood capillaries in the kidney responsible for filtering out waste products. So far, so good. Now, how does this relate to CKD?

It is considered the best indication of measuring kidney function when used as part of a formula that includes age, gender, body size, race and serum creatinine level. Creatinine is a waste product of muscle activity. What actually happens is that our bodies use protein to build muscles and repair themselves. This used protein becomes an amino acid which enters the blood and ends up in the liver where it is once again changed. This time it's changed into urea which goes through the kidneys into the urine.

The harder the muscles work, the more creatinine that is produced and carried by the blood to the kidneys where it also enters the urine. This in itself is not toxic, but measuring the urea and creatinine shows the level of the clearance of the harmful toxins the body does produce. These harmful toxins do build up if not voided until a certain level is reached which can make us ill. Working kidneys filter this creatinine from your blood. When the blood levels of creatinine rise, you know your kidneys are slowing down. During my research, I discovered that a non-CKD patient's blood is cleaned about 35 times a day. A CKD patient's blood is cleaned progressively fewer times a day depending upon the stage of the patient's disease.

In Kathryn Seidick's *Or You Can Let Him Go*, she quotes her son's doctor, "The word you will come to love or dread, Mr. and Mrs. Seidick, is creatinine. This is a substance constantly secreted by muscles, and its presence in the blood shows better than anything how well the kidney is doing. If the creatinine is low, 0.5 to 1.5, the kidney is doing well; if it is high, the kidney is in trouble." This book was published in 1984, but Dr. Gruskin's words are still apt, although he was referring to a child's creatinine levels. A mature man's can be between 0.6 to 1.2, and a mature woman's between 0.5 and 1.0. It can be even lower for children and, as you age, it lowers even more. The more websites I visited, the more variation [albeit very slight] I noticed in acceptable ranges for non-CKD creatinine levels.

DaVita has an estimated GFR calculator on its website at: http://www.davita.com/tools/gfr-calculator/#. However, you will need your serum creatinine reading to use it. There is more information here that I cannot explain than I can since I'm not a medical professional. Basically, you enter your information and then a CKD stage comes up. Try it if you're willing to forego understanding the medical terminology.

I decided to trust that my doctor would understand the necessary formula, especially when I saw that mathematical formula, but decided to give the DaVita site calculator a try, too. Sure enough, using the information from my blood test for the creatinine, my information placed me at Stage 3 CKD. When I lost weight, I was placed at Stage 2. It's apparent that this may be the calibration system my doctor uses since it takes body weight into account. There are many other systems that do the same thing. Just looking on the internet will give you an idea of how many and how they differ slightly from each other.

Notice the radio buttons asking if you are Afro-American. Not only are Afro-Americans at higher risk of CKD, but they have higher muscle mass, so the calculation result has to be multiplied by 1.2 for a true reading. That struck me as odd, not the need to re-calculate, but that you can find a true reading for an estimated value.

In 2002, which is not all that long ago, CKD was divided into five stages by the National Kidney Foundation, dependent upon your GFR results. Serum creatinine is used in this formula as well as age, race and gender.

One of the jobs of the kidneys is to remove this muscle activity waste product from your blood. The higher the levels of this in your blood, the lower the kidney function.

Stage 1	90 ml/min or higher	normal or higher
Stage 2	60-89 ml/min	mild
Stage 3	30-59 ml/min	moderate
Stage 4	15-29 ml/min	severe
Stage 5	less than 15 ml/min	end stage

CKD progresses slowly. Using these divisions, your nephrologist knows how to treat your illness. Each stage requires different treatment. I'll use Stage 2, the stage my tests show, as an example. Usually, at this stage, there are no symptoms. I found out I had CKD when I was being tested for liver function. That's how most people at this stage will be diagnosed: being tested for some other ailment. The blood test I took included GFR estimated routinely. It had never mattered before. Such a test might show up more urea in the blood or, when the urine is tested, protein or blood in the urine. Sometimes, a CAT scan, ultrasound, MRI or contrast X-ray may catch kidney damage. Once diagnosed, you've got to continue monitoring the progress of this disease. I take a blood test and give a random urine sample [that's the pee in a cup kind] once a year and six months later, another blood test accompanied by a 24 hour urine test and give another random urine sample. Other than that, at this early stage, I follow the renal diet [see the next chapter], and try (desperately in my case) to watch my weight including counting calories and exercising daily, whether I want to or not. I should be trying to ingest the Dietary Reference Intake or DRI for vitamins and minerals, but find I often rely on my daily vitamin to do that. If I were a smoker, I would have had to stop. Come to think of it, I was a social smoker, but I think it wouldn't be fair to tell you how easy it was to quit since I only smoked maybe a pack a month.

I am careful about my blood pressure. Right now, my nephrologist and I, working as a team, are checking it twice a day. That means he tells me to take a reading at 10 a.m. and before dinner at 6 p.m. daily with my home blood pressure equipment and I do it. I found my equipment right in the pharmacy and was surprised that it was both a good brand and not too expensive. I've noticed when I'm ill [UTI, flu, etc.], my blood pressure is higher. When I'm not, it's usually within range, which is about 130/85 for me since I have neither diabetes nor proteinuria. The nephrologist and I are actually watching for low blood pressure since it was too low before my HBP medication was cut in half.

My nephrologist is treating me for one aspect of Stage 3. It seems I'm not producing enough Vitamin D, so I now take more Vitamin D supplements. I need this to insure that my bones and teeth remain strong. But, then again, every time I take a blood test, something in my regime is changed because I'm either overloaded with whatever it is or not producing enough of whatever it is. My nephew-in-law calls this my balancing act. He's right. It is all about keeping in balance.

I know there's no cure for CKD, but I'm becoming more and more confidant that I will be able to slow its progress for a long, long time. Brag time: for the first time since I was diagnosed, all my blood tests came back normal. The only downside to that is the test was for an infection which did show up in the urinalysis. I'm still in my positive mode, so I'm sure I'll conquer that, too.

CHAPTER 8:

The Renal Diet

In my research, I found information that amazed me. Apparently, the majority of the U.S. population over 50 suffers from hypertension which may lead to CKD. How are all these people paying for their nutritionist if they do develop CKD, I wondered. Most people think of a nutritionist as a luxury even if they do have a chronic disease. When I pulled out my checkbook to pay my renal dietitian [RD], I was told the government will pay for her services. That made sense. Especially in the current economic atmosphere and for older people, the government needs to help pay our medical bills.

Crystal Barraza, the RD in my nephrologist's Arizona Kidney Disease & Hypertension Center practice, clarified the reasoning behind the diet with the following:

> One of the most obvious messages [I've heard] is that when people are sick, the last thing they want to hear is what they can and cannot eat. It makes sense. I feel that this is also true for many who have many chronic illnesses. I have heard, time and time again from patients like you, 'I am not going to be able to eat anything!' My goal for any session is to help destress people about the diet and help with better food choices. The main goal is to help protect your kidney(s). My

favorite word is moderation. I don't feel that eliminating favorite food from anyone's diet is going to help anyone. It has to be realistic for all. So, I have learned that the best approach is to meet you where you are.

In order to fully understand the renal diet, you need to know a little something about electrolytes. There are the sodium, potassium, and phosphate you've been told about and also calcium, magnesium, chloride and bicarbonate. They maintain balance in your body. This is not the kind of balance that helps you stand upright, but the kind that keeps your body healthy. Too much or too little of a certain electrolyte presents different problems. Eating a larger portion than suggested in the renal diet of a low sodium, phosphate, protein or potassium food is the equivalent of eating a high sodium, phosphate, protein or potassium food. This simply did not occur to me until I read it in one of my sources.

Sodium is pretty well known since news articles about its effects have produced an influx of low sodium foods in supermarkets. Too little sodium can be a problem. Since most adults easily consume the estimated required minimum daily 500 mg. without adding salt to food, it's not a common problem. However, excessive sodium intake is. It can lead to hypertension which can be a cause of CKD. It also may lead to edema, or swelling, another possible problem with CKD.

What makes it worse is that there is no internal mechanism that tells us if we need more or less salt. CKD sufferers are in a spot because the kidneys are the only route by which to eliminate excess salt.

Basically, sodium balances fluid levels outside your cells. You need it because it is responsible for watering your cells. This watering is the prompt for potassium to dump waste [cell process by-products] from your cells. Sodium does deal with other functions of the body, but this is a pretty important one.

If you have damaged kidneys and cannot excrete most of the sodium you ingest, you're up against higher blood pressure which may worsen your CKD which may further cut down on your elimination of sodium and so on and so forth in an ever spiraling cycle. In addition, for CKD patients, too much sodium causes fluid retention, thereby causing swelling, further resulting in weight gain, leading to shortness of breath. That's why your nephrologist asks if you've experienced shortness of breath.

That's also why the following are not on the renal diet or, if they are, it is suggested they be eaten in severely limited quantities once in a great while: pizza, frankfurters, canned soup, frozen dinners, luncheon meats, cheese and smoked or cured food. There are low sodium cheeses but you have to search for them. The most common are Swiss and provolone. I had mistakenly thought nitrates were the problem with frankfurters. Although there are now no nitrate brands, they are still too high in sodium.

It's also become possible to buy reduced or no sodium mayonnaise, baking powder, butter, margarine, seasonings and snacks such as crackers, cookies, pretzels and chips. Don't go too far and use salt substitutes. Rather than help, they'll hurt. They contain potassium chloride which could raise your potassium levels.

Another potential problem concerns both salt and water. If these are retained, you develop edema of the soft tissues of the body. Due to gravity, this occurs in the ankles and feet during the day and the back at night. Edema is dangerous if it occurs in the lungs. Restricting salt [sodium] and making use of a **diuretic** to cause the kidneys to increase their output of both sodium and water can cure the problem, but as a CKD patient, consult your nephrologist before you take action.

Too much sodium can also increase your need for potassium. Potassium is something you need to limit when you have CKD despite the fact that potassium not only dumps waste from your cells but also helps the kidneys, heart and muscles to function normally. Too much potassium can cause irregular heartbeat and even heart attack. This can be the most immediate danger of not limiting your potassium. Some of the highly limited foods are my favorites such as chocolate, caffeine, and chips.

Keep in mind that as you age (you already know I'm in my 60s), your kidneys don't do such a great job of eliminating potassium. So, just by aging, you may have an abundance of potassium. Check your blood tests. 3.5-5 is considered a safe level of potassium. You may have a problem if your blood level of potassium is 5.1-6, and you definitely need to attend to it if it's above 6. Speak to your nephrologist (although he or she will probably bring it up before you do).

The National Kidney Foundation is one of the many places that offer a list of the amounts of potassium in certain foods. Here's a little piece of information you might enjoy: neither gin nor whiskey is high in potassium, but wine is. Not being a drinker, I don't see this as important, but then again, alcohol is something CKD patients are supposed to avoid, not totally eliminate.

I found myself in exactly the opposite position: too little potassium with no reasoning behind it. Maybe I'd been a bit too conscientious about draining the liquid from the canned fruits and vegetables I ate which is one way of avoiding potassium. I'd also been really careful about not having lots of low potassium foods at one time since that increases the amount of potassium you're ingesting even though they are low potassium foods.

The nephrologist handed me a list of low, medium and high potassium foods and simply told me to eat more foods on the medium list. I did, drank some of the liquid from the canned fruits I ate and served myself larger portions of low potassium foods. That seemed to solve the problem. Had I been doing too good a job of limiting potassium rich foods? Before this, I'd been missing bananas, the one food I craved during both my pregnancies. When I needed to raise my potassium, I ate one and was surprised to discover it was the aroma, not the taste, which I had missed.

I have to admit I didn't know anything about **phosphorous**. This is the second most plentiful mineral in the body and works closely with the first, calcium. Together, they produce strong bones and teeth. 85% of the phosphorous and calcium in our bodies is stored in the bones and teeth. The rest circulates in the blood except for about 5% that is in cells and tissues. Again, phosphorous is important for the kidneys since it filters out waste via them. Phosphorous balances and metabolizes other vitamins and minerals including vitamin D which is so important to CKD patients. As usual, it performs other functions, such as getting oxygen to tissues and changing protein, fat and **carbohydrate** into energy.

Be aware that kidney disease can cause excessive phosphorus. And what does that mean for Early Stage CKD patients? Not much if the phosphorous levels are kept low. Later, at Stages 4 and 5, bone problems including pain and breakage may be endured since excess phosphorous means the body tries to maintain balance by using the calcium that should be going to the bones. There are other consequences, but this is the one most easily understood.

Milk and diary products contain phosphorous, which is why I'm limited to 4 ounces daily. Other foods that I, for one, need to limit or avoid due to their high phosphorous level are colas, peanut butter (which I, unfortunately, had just discovered much to my delight before being diagnosed), nuts, and cheeses. To give you an idea why, my phosphorous limit per day is 800 mg. Two pancakes contain 476 mg. or well over half my daily allotment. Although both IHOP and Village Inn now make their pancakes from scratch, it's very rarely that I spend so much of my phosphorous allotment on them.

So, why is protein limited? One reason is that it is the source of a great deal of phosphorus. Another is that a number of nephrons were already destroyed before you were even diagnosed. Logically, those that remain compensate for those that are no longer viable. The remaining nephrons are doing more work than they were meant to. Just like a car that is pushed too hard, there will be constant deterioration if you don't stop pushing. The idea is to stop pushing your remaining nephrons to work even harder in an attempt to slow down the advancement of your CKD. Restricting protein is a way to reduce the nephrons' work.

Your kidneys have about a million nephrons, which are those tiny structures that produce urine as part of the body's waste removal process. Each of them has a glomerulus or network of capillaries. This is where the blood from the renal artery is filtered. The glomerulus is connected to a renal tubule, something so small that it is microscopic. The renal tubule is attached to a collection area. The blood is filtered. Then the waste goes through the tubules to have water and chemicals balanced according to the body's present needs. Finally, the waste is voided via your urine to the tune of 50 gallons of fluid filtered by the kidneys DAILY. The renal vein uses blood vessels to take most of the blood back into the body.

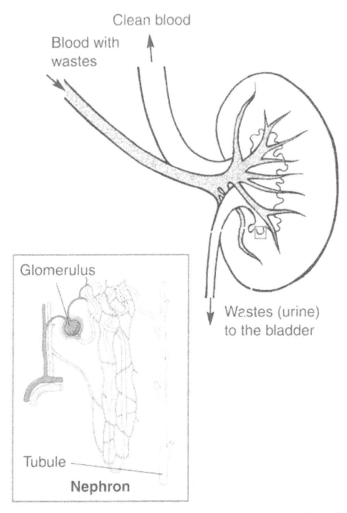

Clean blood

Blood with
wastes

Glomerulus

Wastes (urine)
to the bladder

Tubule

Nephron

*National Institute of Diabetes and Digestive and Kidney
Diseases, National Institutes of Health.*

Keep in mind that there will be times when you'll
need to eat more iron containing foods. Anemia would be
one reason for doing so. There are diets for this and, to
keep it simple, lists of foods and the amount of iron they
contain. You can use the library, ask your nutritionist or
surf the internet for this information. The list I down-

loaded contained so many foods on my no-no list that I wondered how I could bring up my iron level as the nephrologist told me to do.

I looked at my list again, more carefully this time. Okay, there were some foods I could eat and did like on this list. I'm not much for forcing myself to eat food that is distasteful to me. I found beef, which I like only sporadically, shrimp, oatmeal, tuna, chicken, spaghetti (although one cup of this uses up half my starch allotment per day), rice, broccoli and raisins which I consider my candy. I would have to watch the amounts I ate daily, but I could make certain to eat some of these foods each day without thinking of them as medicinal.

When I developed a kidney stone, I was introduced to the **purine** diet. I liked the thought that, yet again, I could medicate myself via food instead of drugs. The idea was to limit the uric acid levels in your blood and urine. This uric acid is produced by purines. Although dietary restrictions are helpful, the body also produces purines. The only foods I needed to avoid that I liked were mushrooms, green peas, berries, concord grapes and oatmeal. Oatmeal is a good source of iron so even if I needed more iron, it would have to come from other foods since I had to limit the purines I ingested. So you see, it's constantly a battle to balance whatever your body needs at the time. It might be oatmeal when you have low iron levels or no oatmeal if you have kidney stones or gout.

I follow the Northern Arizona Council on Renal Nutrition Diet that my nutritionist helped to review and edit. I also looked at several other renal diets to find commonalities so that I'm not describing one diet over all others.

Someone remarked when I mentioned I was on a renal diet that they were all overwhelming and depressing. I'm not sure why he mentioned depressing, unless he meant the restrictions on the goodies. As for overwhelming, yes, it was at first, but the taste buds do adapt and you can find ways to combine the food on the diet so that it is palatable. There are so many cookbooks with meals created for the renal patient.

AAKP has a nutrition counter on their website. It gives the portion size, sodium, potassium, phosphorous, protein and calorie count of a myriad of foods. There are alphabetical radio buttons at the top of the page so you need not scroll through the alphabet to find a specific food. Some popular restaurants, such as IHOP, also have nutritional information on their website, but it's not common to find sodium, potassium or phosphorous listed there.

I'm pretty happy with a handful of this or a handful of that. By this, I mean I measure my servings but don't necessarily mix them to cook. For example, I'll grab 1/3 cup of carrots rather than cook up a whole meal, or I'll put a turkey burger in the toaster oven, slap a potato bread bun around it and call it dinner. That's two starch units and two of the five ounces of protein. Eating this way, sometimes I'm hard-put to include all three servings of vegetables, three of fruit, five ounces of protein and six starches, not to mention fats and dairy during a single day.

I was also assured I'd memorize this stuff easily. I didn't believe it. That involved numbers. I was sure I couldn't memorize numbers. But I did, somewhat. Not only can I now eyeball the servings of each category and keep a list of how many servings of each category I've eaten that day, but some of the calorie counts have stuck with me, too. I'm surprised and delighted that after two years, I don't need to constantly pull out my permissible foods and serving size bible or the calorie counter. I also strictly measured portions for the first two years.

I need to amend something. I thought I could eyeball amounts per serving, but now I'm beginning to wonder. There's that unexplained weight gain despite the exercising and counting calories. Ohhhh, sometimes it hurts to be so brutally honest with yourself, but I'd prefer that pain to curtailing my life by being dishonest with myself.

The diets seem to agree that protein, sodium, phosphorus and potassium need to be limited. I find it easier to remember them if I refer to them as "the three peas with salt." I know it's silly, but it works for me. Apparently, your limits may be different from mine or any other patient's. In other words, it's personalized. Based on my lab results, my potassium limits were raised, so it looks like your limits have a great deal to do with your lab results. Weight is another factor that has to be taken into account. Someone who weighs more than I do (I'm sure such people exist, really), would probably have higher limits than I do.

Although your renal diet is somewhat the same as every other CKD patient's, there are variations. They have to do with the results of your last blood test [hence, the adjustment for low potassium in mine], age, body mass, gender, lifestyle, eating habits and food preferences which your nutritionist will be asking about at your initial meeting, and your general health outside of your CKD.

Again, based on my particular body, I am taking cranberry, calcium and iron supplements. They work for me. They may not work for you. For example, I had been taking 500 mg. of calcium three times a day. Then a teeny, little kidney stone was uncovered. I had no effects from it and was unaware of its existence until it showed up on a sonogram that was ordered for another problem. Calcium supplements could contribute to kidney stones, so now I take the 500 mg. only twice a day.

Herbal supplements can be a problem, too, since only a few have been studied with CKD patients. Keeping in mind that my kidneys are not functioning up to snuff, I decided to abandon them completely. This was quite a departure from the way I usually dealt with illness, but I was frightened enough to just stop using them. I also didn't know if any of them contained "the three peas with salt" or phosphorous, protein, potassium or sodium. I wasn't willing to accidentally further damage my precious kidneys.

While none of this is established, the following might be toxic to the kidneys - wormwood, periwinkle, sassafras (I remember drinking sassafras tea as a child. Did that have any effect on my kidneys?) and horse chestnut just to name a few. Then there are the herbal supplements that might be harmful to CKD patients: alfalfa, aloe, bayberry, capsicum, dandelion, ginger, ginseng, licorice, rhubarb and senna. There are others, but they seemed too esoteric to include. I found I was continuing to learn information that had nothing to do with CKD, but was surprising none the less. For instance, I'd always used a broken open aloe stalk to treat burns never once realizing it was ingestible.

While I urge you to speak with your nephrologists before eating any of these, there are several websites that may be helpful. They are www.herbalgram.org and www.nccam.nih.gov. And, as my nutritionist kept mentioning, star fruit is toxic for CKD patients. Gulp! I ate that, too, when I was in Nigeria. Again, I feel like the medical student who was convinced she suffered from every illness she studied, except in my case, I think everything I ate that's not good for CKD patients was the cause of my disease.

Most of the renal diets limit liquid intake daily, despite the fact that humans lose one liter of water through our skin daily via evaporation. We also lose fluid through breathing, sweating and feces. Men are 60% fluid, which includes not only water but blood and salvia while females are 55% fluid. The kidneys are the organs responsible for regulating the fluids in our bodies.

As CKD patients, we do not internally control the amount of liquid in our bodies, so we have to do it externally. If we drink too little or sweat too much, we become dehydrated. Severe dehydration can cause sweating, diarrhea, vomiting and usually the low blood pressure that makes you feel weak and dizzy when you stand up. On the other hand, if we drink too much, we suffer fluid overload.

It's thirst that makes us drink in order to dilute the concentration of dissolved solids in our bodies so we can bring them back to the proper level. Unfortunately, the brain concurrently releases vasopressin, which is an anti-diuretic hormone that causes the kidneys to conserve water. What this means is that those of us with CKD drink when we've thirsty as does everyone else, but we don't produce much concentrated urine.

If you fall below the proper concentration of dissolved fluids, normally you lose interest in drinking while your urine becomes diluted and you void a great deal of it. However, if you suffer from CKD, there's little increase in urine flow and the urine doesn't become diluted. In other words, a person with CKD – like you or me – has a low concentration of dissoluble solids.

I've already mentioned that my fluid intake restriction is 64 ounces and that I drink two eight ounces cups of coffee daily (I think they help to keep me from feeling deprived), so I'm left with only 48 ounces of liquid. In researching for this book, I discovered that the organic soy milk I sometimes have with cold cereal in the morning and the ice cream I sometimes have are considered fluids as well as being considered dairy.

I don't have both on the same day since my allotment is only four ounces of dairy. That's only half a cup. Have you ever tried to enjoy a quarter cup of ice cream? That's what I'd have to do as well as limit myself to two ounces of that soy milk to enjoy (hah!) them both on the same day.

Going back to the fluid intake, between the coffee and the dairy, I only have 44 ounces of fluid left per day. I live in Arizona where the summer temperatures go up to 115 degrees. I've learned to plan when I'm going to have water and how little to have each time. You'll have to do the same depending upon the climate. This is one time when that old dieting adage which recommends drinking water instead of eating whenever you think you're hungry is not apt, and it's certainly not necessary to drink when others do just to be social.

You might need to be reminded that popsicles, sherbet and gelatin are also fluids, though in solid form. You might need to be reminded, but I needed to learn that. To me, a solid was a solid and a liquid was a liquid. But that's not true for CKD patients. Think about it. Popsicles and sherbet are frozen water with flavoring (I know I'm being too simplistic here.) and gelatin is boiled water with a powder added. This certainly made me curious about what else I didn't know about what I always thought I knew.

My fiancé made us a treat today: strawberry smoothies which consisted of the ½ cup of strawberries that can comprise one of my three fruit units today and four ounces of vanilla ice cream or my one and only dairy unit for the day. I count this as a fruit and a dairy, but should it also be considered part of my remaining 48 ounces of liquid? This is the type of quandary I run into in one form or another on a daily basis. As already mentioned, dairy is, indeed, taken into account as part of your fluids.

As a non-drinker and someone who doesn't care for soda, I had no problem eliminating those from my diet, but my beloved hot chocolate is something I now have maybe once a year. Vitamin and flavored water were just becoming popular when I was diagnosed and, I was surprised to note they are high in sodium, potassium and/or phosphorous.

The list of what to avoid included so many surprises (to me) and the list of beverages that was permitted was so unappealing to me that I'm perfectly content sticking to filtered, non-iced water and coffee. When I go out to dinner unexpectedly, if I've already had my two cups of coffee, I just order hot water and lemon. In over two years, maybe one waiter has asked me to repeat that order.

I was having a dismal time adding up how much sodium, potassium, protein and phosphorous I eat each day although I'd pretty much memorized my allotted food units and the calorie counts of each of my usual foods. I don't know if this is a subconscious revolt against all the bookkeeping or if I truly was incapable of keeping this all straight. My son-in-law told me that eventually food packages will have bar codes containing how much of each of these is in it and our phones will be able to read these labels for us. I sure hope he wasn't kidding.

I devised a little notebook as the CKD patient's food helper. My nephrologist gave me a printed copy of the AAKP Nutrition Counter. This can also be downloaded from their website, but this one was already printed and collated. It measured four inches high by five and a half inches wide. At about the same time, I found a notebook of three by five inch ruled index cards. That was a close enough match for me to realize I could tape the nutrition counter in the back of the notebook and make life easier for myself. I managed to get a week's worth of counting calories, food units, and elements on the front and back of one index card.

I listed each food unit I ate that day and circled the unit [e.g. dairy, protein, etc.] when I reached my limit for the day. Each time I ate something, I used the nutrition counter in which food is listed alphabetically and contains portion size for the elements and calories. I just now am beginning to be able to quickly tabulate the amount of each element and calories in the food and keep a running total until I'd reached my limit for the day. It is cumbersome, but I hope to get it down to a science. Then it will become second nature, just as counting food units and calories has become. If I don't routinely pull this little helper out at the start of a meal, my daughter automatically asks me where it is. It's actually becoming part of who I am. I have high hopes for this helper.

Sample (Unrealistically Neat) Page from An Earlier Notebook Entry

Monday			Tuesday	Wednesday
2 coffee	458	1500NA	**2 coffee**	30
3 fruit	757	3050K	6 starch	383
2 veg.	<u>150</u>	612 P	**5 protein**	20
5 protein	987	750 PRO	dairy	134
1 starch			2 veg.	134
dairy			1 fruit	34
				3
				121
				8
				19
				<u>154</u>
				1040

The first column for the day (shaded) is the food group column in which I recorded the number of units of the food I'd eaten from each group. I've shaded these lists so you can easily locate them. In order to make this neat enough to read, I've used bold lettering [rather than the circles I actually used in my notebook] to indicate when I'd reached my daily limit for that food group. The groups are listed in the order I ate the first food in that group that particular day. On each day, coffee – not a food group but limited, so included – was the first thing I had. Then I ate fruit next on Monday, but starch next on Tuesday. By looking at the food unit column, I could also see where I was falling down. For example, I ate only two portions of vegetables each day. I knew I needed to increase that number to three on the following days.

The second column is a calorie count. You can see that on Monday, I was neither rushed nor tired so I could mentally add quite a few of the individual calorie counts of the food I ate and you only see a few numbers with the grand total on the bottom [458, 757, 150 = 987]. Tuesday, a teaching day, was far busier for me so I needed to write down even the three calories of a bite of something or other. It was easier to write it down as soon as I could and total it later. Naturally, as you can see from the length of the calorie count column, the number next to the food does not necessarily correspond to that food.

I needed to take into account my limitations on protein, potassium, phosphorous, and sodium – three peas with salt. On Monday, you see 1500NA. That's sodium. My limit for this was 2000 mg. per day, so I did all right on Monday. K is potassium which is limited to 3000 mg. daily for me. Uh-oh, I didn't do so well with potassium that day. P equals phosphorous of which I could have 800 mg. per day, so those 612 mg. were not a problem. Although protein is one of the food groups, there are also grams of protein in other foods, so you need to keep account of how many mg. you have a day in addition to how many units of the protein food group you eat each day. Since my limit for protein is five ounces a day which equals 35 grams [one ounce of meat is about seven grams], my 60 gram limit on protein is fairly generous. By the way, all these different limits are based on your individual weight and nutritional needs.

You can see that I didn't fill in the elements for Tuesday. I kept a running list of the foods I ate on the back of my notebook intending to figure out the amounts of each element in those foods when I got home. That was not a good idea since I forgot to do it. That was also the last time I tried that, and I do not suggest you try it.

Not only is my sample notebook page unrealistically neat, but it took much more room to type it out neatly than it actually takes when handwritten. That's why you can fit an entire week's worth of this sort of accounting on the front and back of one index card of your notebook.

I kept refining the way I kept the notebook and playing around with different options, but this straight forward method was the one that worked the best for me. Depending upon your mathematical ability, you may just choose to run all the totals in your head. Or, conversely, you may choose not to keep a single tally mentally. The choice is yours.

CHAPTER 9:

Other Medical Issues When You Have CKD

Your kidneys are compromised. That has a bearing on every infection, cold, surgery, disorder or anything else medical that may happen during your life. You need to be careful about any prescription drugs you may take. You need to read the accompanying literature very carefully to look for **interactions**. You have to read this material every time you obtain a refill since there may be new information about the drug since the last time you filled a script.

The idea is to be vigilant about prescribed drugs that may create some kind of side effect which may further damage your kidneys. It's a good idea to make certain your pharmacist knows you have CKD. Naturally, you need to inform your nephrologist of any medications you intend to start or stop taking.

A case in point is erythropoietin [EPO]. This may be prescribed for anemia. The kidneys produce this protein which promotes the creation of red blood cells. A low red blood cell count may indicate anemia. Your liver also produces a small amount of EPO. All right, let's say you're not producing enough EPO and develop anemia. Your nephrologist prescribes EPO injections.

However, EPO can worsen your HBP - which can both cause and be caused by CKD. Most nephrologists agree it's better to take the EPO injections and increase your HBP medication to control your hypertension. Incidentally, low blood pressure is less serious than high blood pressure, but it still must be treated.

I'll use my own situation as an example of how carefully CKD patients need to monitor their own health. I had a bladder infection, but didn't know it. I knew I wasn't feeling well at all, so I called my primary care physician for an appointment. Her medical assistant [**M.A.**] told me my doctor was out of town for a week and to go to the urgent care center near my home since, as a CKD patient, I should not wait. When I told the receptionist at the urgent care center that I had CKD, she sent me to the emergency room at the local hospital in case I needed blood tests or scans for which the urgent care center was unequipped. The hospital did run a scan and blood tests. This way, they were able to see if I had an infection, blockage or some imbalance that might not only make me feel sick but worsen the CKD.

I already knew I had a higher than usual white blood cell count from my previous fasting blood test for the nephrologist about a month before the emergency room visit. He'd felt it was not significantly high enough to indicate an infection but was, rather, a function of a woman's anatomy. Women have shorter internal access to the bladder, as opposed to those of men. Looked like my nephrologist might have misjudged.

However, he quickly picked up that the medication prescribed by the emergency room physicians, despite my having reiterated several times that I have CKD, was a sulfur based drug. He quickly made a substitution, saving possible further damage to my kidneys. The hospital insisted I only had Stage 2, so this was a safe drug for me. I was nervous about this as soon as they became defensive about prescribing this medication. You need to stick to your guns about being taken seriously when it comes to CKD.

I have had non-nephrology doctors tell me ridiculous things such as there's nothing wrong with an Advil here or there or that I needed more then five ounces of protein a day. I used to argue with them until I realized that I am the one responsible for slowing down the deterioration of my kidneys. I have the help of my nephrologist and nutritionist, but it is ultimately up to me not to blindly listen to a doctor's orders. I need it explained, I need to understand if this is safe for me, and most importantly, I need to speak up if I feel it is not. You, too, need to be your own advocate. Take a friend with you to your appointments if you need moral support, but do not let anyone – doctor or not – dictate to you.

Of course, you already know about not taking non-steroidal anti-inflammatory drugs [**NSAIDS**] like Advil, Aleve and Ibuprofen, much less aspirin which can have an effect on your blood's clotting ability possibly causing bleeding and harming the kidneys. But did you know that certain other over the counter remedies can also be harmful to your health as a CKD patient?

They may contain elements you should not be taking if you have CKD. For example, Alka Seltzer or baking soda is high sodium, and you are already trying to control your sodium intake. Then there are antacids which may contain milk of magnesia, which can build up in your body and cause neurological difficulties. Food supplements or vitamins may contain potassium or magnesium. Even diuretics can damage your kidneys by causing excess sodium excretion. Read the labels and, if you're not sure, ask your nephrologist. As I discovered, it's better to be a pain in that doctor's neck than risk taking a perfectly ordinary substance that had become a threat to you since your kidneys are not working as they should. It's a good idea to avoid enemas and laxatives since they may dramatically and quickly change your electrolyte balance.

There is a psychological trick to remembering to take your prescribed medication [for CKD or other ailments] in the proper quantity and on time. When it's prescribed, ask exactly what it is for and what it is supposed to do. The simple act of remembering this discussion, picturing your doctor possibly pointing at a diagram, picturing yourself possibly watching your doctor's face, and hearing the words said at the time will keep the medication – and the proper time to take it - in the forefront of your mind.

All CKD patients want that cure, that miracle that is going to rid us of CKD. As of now, it doesn't exist, so be leery of any product that promises to do just that. Remember the old adage: if it sounds too good to be true, it is. I noticed overuse of the following words in the advertisements for such products: secret, breakthrough, quick, guaranteed. My initial reaction is, "Yeah, right," before I navigate away from the site or turn the page in that particular magazine.

On the other hand, complementary and alternative medicine may be helpful. Holistic medicine includes the physical, mental, emotional and spiritual. It seems to me that your nephrologist also deals with the physical, but who is tending to the mental, emotional and spiritual aspects of your health?

Some people may prefer to have a therapist or psychologist tend to their emotional state. Help in any of these areas can only be welcome. Although they are not the kind of treatments taught in medical school, some hospitals and insurance companies do cover these alternative or complementary medicine practices. Check with yours to see if the mental, emotional or spiritual help you want is covered.

Then there's preventative medicine, which is what your nephrologist will probably encourage you to practice anyway. This is the kind of medicine in which you, the patient, are educated to prevent more health problems [renal diet, exercise, etc.] rather than just treating symptoms you already have. It also gives you the information you need to stick to your guns when a physician who doesn't know you is trying to prescribe something you know will do further damage to your kidneys.

You'd be surprised at what was once considered alternative medicine. Once practices have been proven both effective and safe, they become part of mainstream medicine. These include osteopathy [an overly simplistic explanation would be the joining of medical practices and chiropractics], chiropractics, acupuncture, acupressure [more commonly referred to as acupuncture without the needles], diet, hypnosis, music, art, visualization, relaxation, massage, vitamins, and meditation.

In the helpful site, www.nccam.nih.gov., *nih* is part of the address. That means the National Institute of Health, and it's a government site. This may help you decide which of these disciplines interest you. As usual, check with your nephrologist before you act on your decision. You don't want to start something that might either be harmful or undermine your treatment in a way you may not have thought about.

There's also help of another sort - psychological. This doesn't necessarily mean heavy duty therapy. I've found online chat rooms and message boards by entering CKD in a search. I've already mentioned that I'm not the joining kind, but that doesn't mean that I don't get some comfort from lurking on these sites. I've found answers to questions I didn't know I had until I read them. I also was able to identify feelings I had been vaguely aware of when

I found them being discussed on message boards. Sometimes, lurkers - people who observe rather than participate - are invited to join the conversation. Other times, you're left alone until you feel you can join in or leave the site.

There are also live support groups for those who want the eye contact, the hugs, the chance to read body language. Your nephrologist or your local hospital can help you find such a group or you can find their locations by surfing the web. Support groups may also lead you to come to terms with the fact that, for the rest of your life, you need to declare your CKD for most life and insurance policies. A note on Twitter: I see that they are beginning to include support groups, but as of the printing of this book, I haven't seen any for CKD.

I haven't found too much about sex that's different from the problems of non-CKD patients although with this disease there may be a lower sex drive accompanied by a loss of libido and an inability to ejaculate. Usually, these problems start with an inability to keep an erection as long as usual. The resulting impotency has a valid physical, psychological or psycho-physical cause.

Some of the physical causes of impotence, more recently referred to as Erectile Dysfunction [E.D.] for a CKD patient could be poor blood supply since there are narrowed blood vessels all over the body. Or maybe it's leaky blood vessels. Of course, it could be a hormonal disturbance since the testicles may be producing less testosterone and the kidneys are in charge of hormones. Possibly, you're tired from CKD induced anemia. I've just mentioned a few possibilities. The silver lining is that there are almost as many treatments as there are causes.

While E.D. can be caused by renal disease, it can also be caused by diabetes and hypertension. All three are of importance to CKD patients. Sometimes, E.D. is caused by the medications for hypertension, depression and anxiety. But, E.D. can also be caused by other diseases, injuries, surgeries, prostate cancer or a host of other conditions and bodily malfunctions. Psychologically, the problem may be caused by stress, low self-esteem, even guilt to name just a few of the possible causes.

The usual remedies for E.D. can be used with CKD patients, too, but you need to make certain your urologist and your nephrologist work together, especially if your treatment involves changing medications, hormone replacement therapy or an oral medication like Viagra. There are other treatments not mentioned here since I really don't want to make this a chapter about sex. You can research this yourself by searching something like *sex for CKD patients*.

Sometimes, the treatment is as simple as counseling and the cessation of smoking and alcohol. Hmmmm, as CKD patients, we've already been advised to stop smoking and drinking. This is another reason for male CKD patients to do so.

Women with CKD may also suffer from sexual problems, but the causes can be complicated. As with men, renal disease, diabetes and hypertension may contribute to the problem. But so can poor body image, low self-esteem, depression, stress and sexual abuse. Any chronic disease can make a man or a woman feel less sexual.

Some remedies for women are the same as those for men. I discovered through my research that vaginal lubricants and technique, routine, and environment changes when making love, warm baths, massage, and vibrators can help. Again, there are other, more medical treatments.

Common sense tells us that sex or intimacy is not high on your list of priorities when you've just been recently diagnosed. I was obsessed with my revulsion of dialysis and needed to hear over and over again that it was a couple of decades too early to worry about this. I was also tired and didn't know why, just worried that I would always need an afternoon rest period. (Thanks to my nephrologist's directed regime of iron on a daily basis, no more rest periods!) Then I discovered that vaginal strep B can occur in women over 60 with CKD. Luckily for me, if you catch it and treat it early on, it's just an infection that you take antibiotics to kill. If you don't treat it early, you just may be looking at some serious consequences.

Since we're in the early stages of CKD, chances are the sexual problem is not physical other than being tired. I never talked to my nephrologist about sex because I felt there was no reason to, and I had a partner who was willing to work around my rest periods until I had the energy. But, I am convinced, that if I ever do feel I have reason, I would talk to him. I'm older and prefer women doctors for the most part especially when it comes to private matters but this man is the specialist who knows far more than I do about this disease I am struggling to prevent from progressing. There is a point when you realize your life is more important than not being embarrassed.

Sometimes people with chronic diseases can be so busy being the patient that they forget their partners have needs, too. And sometimes, remembering to stay close, really close as in hugging and snuggling, can be helpful. You've got to keep in mind that some CKD patients never have sexual problems, no change in frequency and depth of desire and no impairment in the act itself. This is not the time to make yourself the textbook case of the CKD patient who suffers sexually because of her disease. The best advice I received in this area was make love even if you don't want to. Magic.

One caution for the pre-menopausal women reading this book: use protection even if you think you are incapable of becoming pregnant. Pregnancy is risky for women with CKD. The risks for both the mother and fetus are high as is the risk of complications. You'll need to carefully discuss this with your nephrologist and your gynecologist should you absolutely, positively want to bear a child rather than adopt.

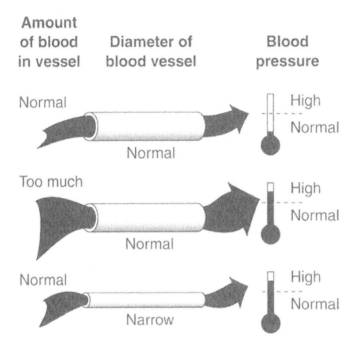

| Amount of blood in vessel | Diameter of blood vessel | Blood pressure |

National Institute of Diabetes and Digestive and Kidney Diseases, National Institutes of Health.

Blood pressure is such an issue with CKD patients that I'm including more information about that here. The diagram above demonstrates how too much blood flowing through a normal or narrow sized artery can cause high blood pressure, while the normal amount of blood flowing through a normal sized artery produces a normal blood pressure reading. You should know first that 31%, or almost one third, of adults over the age of 20 in the United States have HPB with an additional 25% in the pre-hypertensive range. Furthermore, as we age, it's natural for our blood pressure to change. The most up to date figures [August, 2010] show the following guidelines:

Normal blood pressure: **below 120/80**
Pre hypertension [pre HBP]: 120/80 to 139/89
HBP: 140/90 to 159/99
Very HBP: 160/100 or above

You'll notice the two numbers. I'd always been curious about that but either too rushed or too lazy to research what it meant. The first number [shaded], called the systolic is the rate at which the heart contracts, while the second or diastolic [unshaded] is when the heart is at rest between contractions. These numbers measure the units of millimeters of mercury to which your heart has raised the mercy. Contrary to popular belief, headache is not always a sign of HBP just as weakness or dizziness when you stand up is not always a sign of low blood pressure [LBP]. In order to make your HBP medication effective, high cholesterol, obesity and smoking have to be treated simultaneously.

Before you become upset at your own blood pressure reading, you should know that your blood pressure is higher in the morning and early evening, is different between arms and may register differently if you use different equipment or use the same equipment in a different manner. It can also be affected by the percentage of water in your body and the width of your arteries. Narrower arteries can raise your blood pressure [take another look at the diagram on the previous page]. Then there are the minor changes such as white coat syndrome. That's when you become fearful or stressed about what the reading will be in the doctor's office which raises the reading a little bit.

A **sphygmomanometer** measures the pressure of the blood on the artery wall. Humans have 10 pints of blood that are pumped by the heart through the arteries to all the other parts of the body. This oxygen rich blood combines with whatever was eaten to provide energy. Our **veins** move the oxygen depleted blood back to the heart and then the lungs for more of the oxygen you took in by breathing. This is a constant process. If blood pressure is taken against the artery walls, then it's oxygen rich blood that is being measured.

I can't quite figure out if this is good news or bad, but it seems CKD sufferers are more likely to die from the disease's complications rather than the disease itself. You can see this from the list of the most frequent causes of death in people with CKD: infection, stroke, noncompliance with your treatment plan, cancer or (the ubiquitous) unknown. We're getting far, far ahead of ourselves since this book was written for those in the early stages of the disease, but I felt it important for you to know that you can prolong your life by making sure you take care of yourself.

CHAPTER 10:

Getting the Necessary Exercise

I eagerly anticipated writing this book because I didn't fully understand just how all this exercise would be helpful. I knew researching would clarify it in my mind, and it has. But then, a new wrinkle entered my life: I stopped losing weight and even gained a few pounds despite my minimum of a half hour of daily exercise. This while I was strictly adhering to the renal diet, the one that required only a certain number of food units for each food group a day.

I knew exercise was important to control my weight. It would also improve my blood pressure and lower my cholesterol and triglyceride levels. The greater your triglycerides, the greater the risk of increasing your creatinine. There were other benefits, too, although you didn't have to have CKD to enjoy them: better sleep, and improved muscle function and strength. But, as with everything else you do that might impinge upon your health, check with your doctor before you start exercising.

I researched, researched and researched again. Each explanation of what exercise does for the body was more complicated than the last one I read. Keeping it simple, basically, there's a compound released by voluntary muscle contraction. It tells the body to repair itself and grow stronger. The idea is to start exercising slowly and then intensify your activity.

I've been dancing in one form or another since I was eight years old as far as I can remember. Being an independent person, I had trouble following choreographed routines so I couldn't dance in shows (well, that's the reason I gave myself). Later on, as a single mother of two, I had a problem getting to dance lessons since the kids' activities always seemed to fall on my dance class nights.

But they were busy with their own social lives on the weekends, so I could go dancing at the clubs then. That didn't work so well, either, since I was neither a hot young thing who commanded dance partners by my very appearance, nor was I comfortable going into any place that served liquor. I didn't drink myself and had previously had some bad experiences with people who did drink. I did realize it was possible to be a social drinker without drinking to excess, but was already prejudiced against drinking establishments by my prior experiences in them.

As a young woman back in the 1930s, my mother had gone to tea dances with her older brother. These included swing dancing, and she became very, very proficient at this. We always listened to swing music when she came to visit, but I'd never tried to dance to it. Then I found a swing dance class at the local YMCA during the same time my children had their ballet (for one) and singing (for the other) lessons. It was a tight fit time-wise, but I could do it.

I met a single dad there whose son was at Cub Scouts at the same time in the same building. We hit it off as dance partners and decided to try the clubs together. I convinced him that he could meet eligible young ladies there but didn't really know if that were true. We tried some of the swing clubs in New York City and had a great time, but he didn't meet anyone, so we started going to the swing dances instead. Bingo! He met more women than he'd thought he would, I had my dance partner, and

I learned to appreciate dancing with other partners. The swing dances are also much less expensive than the clubs which charge a minimum for drinks whether you drink or not.

Most swing dances don't serve liquor although water is always available. More importantly to me, they are open to people of all ages so I tried to get my kids interested. The ballerina didn't like the beat, and the singer didn't like dancing at all. That's when I started going by myself whenever my daughters had social engagements. The dances weren't meat markets, no liquor was served and there were plenty of dance partners. The whole thing was comfortable for a woman alone and I got to exercise, often vigorously.

What I didn't know at the time is that your body becomes accustomed to a certain kind of exercise and then it isn't as effective anymore. Yes, it was definitely fun, the music always raised my spirit and the dancing created quite a sweat if done correctly, but I was at the point when I needed to find something else in addition.

I was newly diagnosed and had realized swing dancing wasn't enough exercise when my daughter asked me to come back East for two weeks so I could attend the two bridal showers she was having there. While she'd become a swing dancer herself once she grew up, she lived in a remote part of New York with only one dance a month. That one dance wasn't going to be while I was there.

All I could think of was walking at a brisk pace. It worked! I walked all around the rural area where she was living, in the suburbs of New Jersey where the other shower was being held, and in the airports waiting for my planes. I got my heart rate up and the sweat going (sorry, fellow fliers).

I was hooked and walked like this whenever I couldn't dance. I live in Arizona where every swing dance is at least half an hour's travel each way, with most of them being an hour or more away, but I could walk in nearby malls and big box stores when I needed to walk indoors. That was pretty often since the summers are brutal in Arizona.

Then I discovered indoor walking tracks at a local community center. It cost me $5.00 each time I used the local indoor track, but I've since discovered one community center that charges $5.00/year. It's just a matter of using the phone or the internet to locate the less expensive tracks. Most high schools have tracks that are open to the community free of charge when their track teams or physical education classes are not using them. I loaded my iPod with murder mysteries and walked for chapters at a time.

My chosen sister decided to exercise with me once a week to support my efforts and introduced me to Leslie Sansone's walking tapes. I liked them so much that I figured I would do them at home by myself. I found ways to make this more comfortable by buying some inexpensive outdoor playground mats and laying them on the living room floor so my arthritic knees and hips didn't bother me as much. I have tile floors, so this softened the impact of each step.

I also started using knee braces that I found for sale in the pharmacy. They are neither expensive nor do they require script. This exercising was getting easier and easier to do. You've probably figured out that my body got used to this, too. So, I still walk and dance but have added other types of exercise.

As a college instructor, I was entitled to free tuition including physical education classes. What I did was register for the ones held in the fitness center. There was a trainer on the floor at all times and loads of different machines to work different parts of your body as well as stationary bicycles and treadmills. It was here that I learned the value of light weights to intensify your exercise routine without causing undue stress. By researching a little bit, I discovered that soup cans and filled water bottles work just fine as weights if you're not in a position to purchase them. The college fitness center wouldn't allow these, but I did use them at home.

Remember, I was already in my sixties when the CKD diagnosis led to me search for different types of exercise that I like. I knew if I didn't like it, I was bound to start finding excuses not to do the exercise. Now I had swing dancing, walking and the fitness center at my disposal, but I wanted more.

Sometimes I couldn't go to the gym because I wasn't teaching that term and didn't want to pay the full amount to join a gym that was over half an hour away and now required a special trip to campus just to use the fitness center. Sometimes I couldn't dance because my arthritic hip was causing too much pain. Sometimes I couldn't use the walking tapes because the arthritic knee was acting up.

That's when I was introduced to water walking, something I'd never heard off until I relocated to Arizona and met someone who lived in Sun City. Retirement communities out here have their own community centers and members can bring guests. The water walking pool is a gigantic track that is underwater. Directional arrows are painted on the floor of the pool to let you which direction to walk, so you're not walking into other people.

Our temperatures can go as high as 115 degrees so there were days when I just couldn't wait to water walk. It was cool and refreshing, and you were using the water's resistance to burn calories. This year, I got myself water walking gloves which are waterproof gloves with webbing between the fingers. I hold my arms out under the water to increase the water resistance. I have seen people at the pool with water weights, but have not tried that myself yet.

I noticed a bowling alley right next to the pool building. Now that's another way of exercising and having a good time simultaneously. Unfortunately, both my partner and I had shoulder surgery recently so we had to hold off on the bowling for a while. So now, I had swing dancing, walking, water walking and bowling in my exercise arsenal. I was always on the lookout for new forms of exercise that are fun so I'd look forward to them.

Some people enjoy tennis or golf. Before moving to Arizona, I lived on a small island that had municipal courts and greens. They weren't totally free, but so low cost that many people didn't wait for the weekend but went before or after work. Some families with children used these kinds of exercise as a family affair, so they could spend time with the children while getting in their exercise.

There's ice skating, skiing and snow boarding, too. Being arthritic, these are not sports I can participate in comfortably any more, but you might be able to. These are also good bonding experiences for families. I would go with my children and sit in the skate house or lodge, watching them and being there with them whenever they came in to warm up. I can only imagine how much more fun it would be to actually be outdoors with the kids, getting your exercise, too.

My fiancé bought us an exercise bike as a Christmas present a few years back. I had no idea what a prize this would be. I loved movies, any kind, as long as there were no commercial interruptions. With cable television (a must in my area since we live in a valley surrounded by mountains which made for poor reception), I have Movies on Demand. If I have the money that month, I can just order the movies I want to see on the television. If not, I can go to a Redbox kiosk and rent a movie for $1.00 a day.

Then there is our own DVD library. There are also free movies that are offered with cable and, of course, DVDs from the library. We just pointed the exercise bike toward the television and now I ride as many miles as I want for as long as I want while I watch a movie I'm interested in. Most of the time, I'm surprised at how long I've been on the bike.

While I'm mentioning cable, my older daughter just reminded me to include the Discovery Channel's "FitTV," which she often visits. Nima also explained to her dinosaur of a mother, that you can go to their website to view free workouts videos. The URL is: http://fittv. discovery.com/.

For those who enjoy team sports, there's basketball, hockey, soccer or netball. There are, of course, other teams I haven't mentioned. Your local community center, Department of Parks & Recreation's center, or house of worship may sponsor these. If not, you can always use the internet to find teams. When I first moved and didn't have the computer up yet, I looked in the phone book for sporting goods stores. Then I went there and looked at their bulletin boards for announcements of new teams or existing teams looking for new members. Coffee house bulletin boards are another good place to look.

If you're the type that would prefer organized classes, there's yoga, Pilates, karate, step, dance, Qigong, judo, aikido, Krave Maga or just about any other kind of exercise that interests you. You can look for studios that teach these disciplines, schools or – what I found the least expensive – continuing education at the local college or at nearby public schools.

If you're not a joiner, you can always rollerblade, ride your bike outdoors, jog or skateboard. Maybe you'd rather surf or swim. Then again, maybe you'd rather boogie your way through your housework or gardening. As long as you keep moving and burning those calories, you're exercising.

By now, I feel antsy if I haven't gotten my minimum of half an hour of exercise every day, but in the beginning I was very organized. I had a heart rate monitor [you can order one for about $30] and my iPod. I would make a check on the calendar after I'd exercised, so I could get a sense of accomplishment from seeing those check marks. I carried sneakers and socks in the trunk of my car in case it was one of those crazy days when my plans didn't work so well, I was running out of time in the day and hadn't gotten any exercise in yet. That's when I would stop at a mall and do a couple of brisk turns inside.

I've discovered articles that say you need to exercise every day, and those that say you need to take a day or two off each week. Frankly, I'm at the point where I try for every day but remember the articles that say take a day or two off each week if I don't get to make the time every day that week. I don't know if it's a function of age or not, but sometimes the day slips away, and I haven't exercised yet.

For me, planning is important. For example, I'm going dancing tonight, so I know I don't have to stop writing to exercise. Yesterday, I did - so I figured that since I can't sit still at the computer for more than two hours at a time, I'd use the exercise bike and watch a movie during my second computer break. The day before, I had appointments left and right without too much time for myself, so I had my coffee in the morning then used a one mile walking tape. I usually use a three mile tape, but knew time was going to be tight that day and figured one mile was better than no miles.

I've learned from my mistakes that when you plan, you need to include a shower in the time you put aside for exercising. If you're doing it right, you're going to sweat. You might want to exercise first thing some days so you can get the shower out of the way before starting the rest of your day. Other times, you might want to exercise later on [but not too close to bedtime since it may keep you up], so you can just take your shower before turning in.

When I was going to the fitness center at the college, I would teach, exercise, shower, then either teach another class or go on to my next appointment. In all honesty, that became too much for me to do since I was wearing teaching clothes, carried a gym bag with all my gym and shower things and my attaché case. I'm more comfortable exercising at home or as a social occasion. That way, I have my shower and clothes right there in my home or there's no need to shower or change because all the people who exercised with me are just as sweaty.

It really doesn't matter how you do it as long as you exercise. There are days when an arthritic hip prevents me from doing any full body exercise. I make sure no one is watching, then I dance vigorously but only from the waist up. If it's summertime here, I can water walk without too much pain when the arthritis acts up.

The point is that exercise is going to help you impede the progress of your CKD. Learn to at least tolerate exercise, if you can't learn to love it.

CHAPTER 11:

Friends and Family Want to Know

Once I recovered from my initial shock at my diagnosis and then the fear of dialysis, I started talking, and talking, and talking. While this might not be an unusual occurrence for me (alas), all I talked about now was CKD. I waited for someone to ask a question about it, then I pounced setting forth volumes for what required a simple, one sentence explanation. But, basically, people were not really asking me about the illness at all.

They were asking what they, as friends and family, could do to help someone in the early stages of CKD. With all my researching and writing, I thought I didn't really need any more help, so I asked my own friends and family what they thought I needed. While some of the answers were predictable, some were not.

My chosen sister advised me that people need to be told that they have to be patient while I order in restaurants. I pour over the menu looking for acceptable foods prepared in the ways I can eat them. Then I ask a myriad of questions about how many ounces, how many calories, what ingredients are not listed on the menu (beware of Coco's which seems to have a surprising number of unlisted ingredients) and how many calories. I usually spend time asking about substitutions of acceptable foods for unacceptable ones in a meal. While I apologize to the waiter or waitress in advance for all the questions, it had never occurred to me that I ought to be apologizing to my dinner companions, too.

My fiancé thinks that the weighing and measuring of food should be explained. He doesn't really care why I need to do it, but he does want to be sure he can help figure out how much of what I can have at a meal or a snack. Since he does the majority of the cooking at our house, he knows to do the weighing measuring after the food is cooked. Sometimes, he's tired from working all day, but has the patience to wait for me to do the weighing and measuring before we sit down to eat. It takes time and we like to eat when the food is hot. In addition, since I'm so restricted in the amounts I can eat, he shares a meal with me when we go out. By the way, he has lost 50 pounds being helpful to me since I have been diagnosed.

My younger daughter, Abby, is also a swing dancer. She wanted to know just what activities cause fatigue for me and how fast this happens. She lives close by, so we see each other as often as we can. She wanted to make sure to help me catch the fatigue before it was so far gone that I couldn't drive home from wherever we were. When I explained it wasn't a particular activity and it doesn't just drop down on me, she asked me what indications there would be that I was becoming fatigued, so she could wind up whatever we were doing before I was a dish rag. She's pretty used to my sitting and watching for a while as she dances now, instead of my dancing every dance the way I used to.

An actor friend who likes to cook wanted a copy of the renal diet so she knew what to cook for me. Then she suggested I tell her how the food should be cooked, so that I can eat it. She had no trouble changing the menu for me and making sure there was some substitute, permissible food for me if I couldn't eat part of the meal she cooked. This is a woman who has a husband, grown children and a grand-child in her household. She said it's just as easy to cook what I can eat, or if someone else at the dinner really wants a certain something I can't eat, offer a substitute for me as it was to cook any other meal. I never would have asked. I'd just assumed it would be too much trouble.

My older daughter was interested in how much sleep I needed. It's recommended that CKD patients get eight hours a night if possible. She's a singer, so we can be out late at karaoke. Now that she knows, we leave the karaoke site in time for me to get that much sleep. If I don't need to get up early the next day, we can stay later (just like the other kids!). Sometimes, if I do have to get up early, but want to go to karaoke with her anyway, I just excuse myself and take a nap before we go. Mind you, she's from out of state so this is while she's visiting. She's not at all insulted, as she probably would have been had she not asked me about my sleep requirements. I'd never have thought to tell her.

A colleague at the college was surprised to hear me say I was going for a cup of coffee. She felt I should let people know I can have two cups a day because she'd pointedly not been inviting me to the local Paradise Bakery since she knew I couldn't have pastries, but didn't know I could have coffee. I let her know I save one cup for when I finish teaching, so we often have that cup of coffee together now. I would have deprived myself of the joy of being able to talk shop with another English instructor if she hadn't overheard me. Now, I tell friends that I "do" coffee, just like anyone else.

Another writer wanted me to sit in Starbuck's and write with him while we drank cup after cup of coffee one afternoon, a seemingly favorite activity of many writers if I'm to believe what I'm told. When I explained about the coffee restrictions, he asked if I like to walk. He was delighted to hear that I needed half an hour's exercise daily and walking was an activity I liked. He didn't want to write, he wanted to talk about our books. You can catch us walking along the Skunk Creek path several times a week. He said that I should have told him about my need to exercise and we could have started doing this a long, time ago.

A neighbor likes to bake and was, of course, bringing me samples every time she did. She noticed I was uncomfortable when she did this once I was diagnosed and asked why. When I told her, she got upset. Not that I couldn't eat her baking, but that I was sick and she was making life difficult for me (as she phrased it). She didn't know I couldn't eat cookies, cakes or pastries. Now she does and we can enjoy a visit without them, although I love the aromas that waft from her open windows to mine when she bakes. She just doesn't bring me samples. She's not uncomfortable and neither am I. I'm only sorry I didn't think to tell her of both my diagnosis and my food restrictions before she had the opportunity to become upset.

It probably seems that most of what our friends and family want to know deals with food. I think that's true since we can retard the deterioration of our kidneys by watching what we eat, how much we eat, and how it's prepared. Quite a few of their questions dealt with exercise and fatigue since it was made clear these are important issues for CKD patients, too.

Some of them want to know about all those medical tests we take, too. One buddy who lives across the country from me was curious as to why I was doing a 24 Hour Urine Collection and, more importantly to her (and me), could she call me that day. I explained that I stayed in because it was more convenient to have the refrigerator right there and my collection bottle in it. I suggested that she could call whenever she wanted to, but she'd just have to understand if I couldn't answer right then. That's when she told me she'd thought I was giving her the bum's rush when I didn't answer my phone or immediately call her back when I got her voice mail the last time I'd done the 24 Hour Urine Collection. This is my good buddy from childhood, so I was especially sorry she'd felt that way. That's another reason friends and family need to know.

I genuinely didn't know that my friends and family wanted to know this about my life as a CKD patient. I didn't think to tell them. What do you need to tell your friends and family so they understand you better? You can't tell by looking at us that we have CKD, we just act in a peculiar fashion sometimes. Maybe you need to explain why, so they'll be a little more comfortable with this behavior. Patients with terminal issues and their caretakers are urged to ask people for what they need. Maybe we need to learn to ask for what we need, too.

CHAPTER 12:

End Notes

Amazing things have happened since I first began writing this book. I started a blog (http://gailrae.word press.com), so that other people with early stage CKD wouldn't have to wait until this book was published to get the support and the information I've offered here.

After reading the blog, people contacted me with all sort of offers. One wanted to introduce me to a friend of his who was a traditional publisher. Another gave me all the information he had about self publishing. A third asked me to lead the education forum, Kidney Matters, for The Transplant Community Outreach on Facebook. The Chronic Kidney Disease Support Forum and The American Society of Nephrologists began carrying my blog on their Facebook pages.The Renal Support Network and KidneyTimes.com featured one of my articles on their front pages.

What I understand from all this and the rest of it that I didn't list is that people in the early stages of CKD needed a book like this just as I did. I'm not happy I have CKD, but I'm glad I could make the journey even a teensy bit easier for anyone else. For a private person, I've been pretty open about my disease and my life. It helped me accept my diagnosis, something I'd hadn't thought about while writing the book. My hope is that it helps you accept yours.

I've met many other CKD sufferers through the internet and asked if they would share their initial reaction to their diagnosis. Here are only a few of the many who whole-heartedly agreed when they realized the idea was to give comfort to those who were newly diagnosed. Sometimes realizing others were in the same position can help you overcome your own despair.

"When I was diagnosed with CKD in 2009, I was surprised because no other doctor had made this diagnosis.... Well, I said, 'What? Why? How? I don't understand.' He didn't have any answers and I had so many questions for him."

"At first, it was a death sentence and I was in shock. I read all I could on the internet. I have friends who are physicians and they said I should be concerned but not frightened...."

"No one can quite tell me where I got mine from also. Improperly diagnosed with high blood pressure since age 17.... Blood pressure went haywire after a bout of pneumonia at age 34."

"... to be honest, I didn't realize I had CKD as it wasn't explained to me. I had accidentally taken a sheet that I was supposed to give to the front desk people, but didn't know and they didn't ask at the time...."

"After my doctor called me, I couldn't believe it. I cried. I was very shocked. I just found out that I have Stage 3 Kidney Disease. I am devastated.... To tell the truth, I am very afraid."

"Those first few weeks were NOT very nice. I thought I had been handed a death sentence…."

"I was diagnosed in May and it took me a little bit before it hit me…. I had no idea even what it was about so didn't give it any more thought.…For some reason this year I went home and looked up GFR. When I began to realize the significance of declining kidney function, I went back and asked what I could do to slow or stop the decline."

It seems a lot of us didn't know what this was and either remained ignorant long past the time we should have started helping ourselves or were shocked into despair. You are not alone. It's not such a pretty disease, but then again, is any disease? It's not fair that you've got it, but that's life. There's only one thing left to do: keep loving your life and live it well. Anyone want to go swing dancing with me tonight?

CHAPTER 13:

Additional Resources

Please note that inclusion in any of these lists is not an endorsement of the organization or the book, newsletter, or website. You need to make up your own mind about the validity of both the information and/or the author.

Books

Due to the scientific nature or exorbitant prices of CKD books, this is a short list. Remember that end stage CKD books about transplants and dialysis will not be on this list either, making it even shorter. Add to that the outdated (I didn't include anything published before 2000, except novels) CKD books and you have a very, very short list of books.

Coping with Kidney Disease: A 12- Step Treatment Program to Help You Avoid Dialysis. Dr. Mackenzie Walser (John Wiley & Sons, Inc., 2004) The title is a good description of the book's contents. The language is fairly medical. This is only one method of dealing with kidney disease, one treatment plan that is quite different from the one I am familiar with from my own treatment.

Driving Sideways. Riley, Jess. (Ballantine Books, 2008) This is a fanciful work of fiction in which the protagonist feels she is channeling the spirit of her kidney donor.

Kidney at a Glance, The. O'Callaghan, Christopher A., and Barry Brenner. (Blackwell, Inc., 2000) This is a good primer and introduction to what the kidneys are and why they are so important.

Kidney Failure Explained. Stein, Andy, and Janet Wild (Class Health, 2002) This is a clear explanation, but deals with the English system, which I found a bit disappointing since I wanted help available to me here in the United States.

Living Well with Kidney Failure. Auer, Juliet et al. (Class Health, 2004) This is a collection of patients' personal accounts of their dealings with their kidney disease.

Mr. Right and My Left Kidney. Saltzman, Joan (Peripety Press, 2006) This memoir tells a love story which includes a character who suffers kidney failure and transplant and discusses these issues as easily as the author discusses finding love later in life.

100 Questions and Answers about Kidney Disease and Hypertension. Townsend, Raymond R., and Dr. Debbie L. Cohen (Jones and Bartlett Publishers, Inc., 2009) This is exactly what the title indicates and not overly medical in its answers. It covers just about every question I could think of, plus those I hadn't thought of.

Ten Step Diet & Lifestyle Plan for Healthier Kidneys: Avoid Dialysis. Koble, Nina. (Mirasmart Digital Publishing, 2009) This one is more diet oriented, but also not so medical that laymen [those who are not in the medical profession] could not understand it.

DVDs

"Chronic Kidney Disease: Are You at Risk?" (Home Use). Information Television Network. June 23, 2008. Amazon.com

"Living with Chronic Kidney Disease" (Home Use). Information Television Network. July 27, 2006. Amazon.com

"Living with Kidney Disease" (British). Kidney Research UK. http://www.kidneyresearchuk.org/shopping/ living-with-kidney-disease-dvd.php   No release date given.

Discussion Forums

You will need to register, but nothing too personal is required.

DaVita Discussion Forum – www.davita.com/forum/ index.php. There are different topics each with its own discussion forum. They deal with all aspects of CKD from the early stages to dialysis.

Facebook Page: Chronic Kidney Disease (CKD) Discussion Forum http://www.facebook.com/#!/group.php?gid=4729239 5689. This is a good place to find the support you may be looking for. Members range from early stage to transplants.

Facebook Page: Kidney Café - Kidney Disease Awareness and Discussion Forum http://www.facebook.com/group.php?gid=832518606 57. I've noticed quite a bit of activity on this discussion forum the entire time I was writing the book.

Facebook Page: Transplant Community Outreach: Discussion Forum – Kidney Matters http://www.face book.com/topic.php?topic=20094&uid=22202055930 6. This deals with early stage CKD. (I know because I write it.)

Healthboards.com - http://index.healthboards.com/ kidney/. There is a drop down list of a multitude of subjects dealing with CKD on this site. You just point and click.

MedHelp – http://www.medhelp.org/posts/Kidney-Disease-Disorders/Kidney-Problem-Symptoms/show/ 1361333. On this forum, you post your question and others will answer it unlike most of the others where there is free give and take.

National Kidney Foundation - http://www.kidney.org/ nkfmb/forums.cfm?conferenceid=DD4F2231-17A4-8D04-9499C70E025BB8C5 As mentioned, this is an outreach of NKF.

Newsletters

For each of these newsletters, you'll need to register your e-mail address.

Health.com - http://news.health.com/category/chronic-kidney-disease/feed/

Mayo Clinic - http://www.mayoclinic.com/health/kidney-failure/DS00682

Medline Plus - http://www.nlm.nih.gov/medlineplus/kidneyfailure.html

National Kidney Foundation - http://www.kidney.org/news/newsletters.cfm

Organizations

American Association of Kidney Patients (AAKP)
3505 E. Frontage Rd., Suite 315
Tampa, Fl. 33607
(800) 749–2257
www.aakp.org

American Kidney Fund (AKF)
6110 Executive Blvd., Suite 1010
Rockville, Md. 20852
(800) 638-8299
www.kidneyfund.org

American Medical Association (AMA)
515 N. State Street
Chicago, IL 60654
(800) 621-8335
www.ama-assn.org

American Society of Nephrology
1725 I Street, NW
Suite 510
Washington, DC 20006
(202) 659-0599
www.asn-online.org

National Kidney Disease Education Program
3 Kidney Information Way
Bethesda, Md. 20892
(866) 454-3639
www.nkdep.nih.gov

National Kidney Foundation (NKF)
30 East 33 St.
NYC, NY 10016
(800) 622–9010
www.kidney.org

National Kidney and Urologic Diseases Information
    Clearinghouse (NKUDIC)
3 Information Way
Bethesda, Md. 20892–3580
(800) 891-5390
www.kidney.niddk.nih.gov

Statistics

Unfortunately, the statistics are not as current as I'd
hoped they'd be. According to Centers for Disease Control
and Prevention, there are approximately 26 million adults
with CKD in the United States. Notice that children are
not included in this number. During 2006, the year these
statistics were released, CKD was the ninth leading cause of
death in the U.S., claiming almost 45,000 lives.

By the next year, Kidney and Urologic Disease Statistics for the United States listed the number of fatalities
from kidney disease at 87,812. This organization counted
527,283 patients under treatment for kidney disease in
2007.

Websites

Note: .gov = government site; .org = organization site; .com = for profit site

Administrators in Medicine's doctor finder. http:// docboard.org

The Agency for Healthcare Research and Quality. Includes insurance choices and clinical trial practice guidelines. [Technical, you may need a medical dictionary.] http://www.ahcpr.gov

Amazon. An online book store for textbooks, biographies, children's books, medical books, cookbooks, treatment plans, educational books. Look for DVDs, videos, audio recordings, e-books and Kindle products, too. http://www.Amazon.com

American Association of Kidney Patients. Renalife, a quarterly kidney magazine, is from this organization. http://www.aakp.org

American Board of Medical Specialties. You can check your doctor's **certification** on this site. https://www. abms.org/wc/login.aspx

American Botanical Council. www.herbalgram.org

American Kidney Fund. http://www.kidneyfund.org

The American Kidney Fund. http://www.akfinc.org

American Medical Association. http://www.ama-assn.org

American Medical Association. A doctor finder. http://webapps.ama-assn.org/doctorfinder/home.jsp

American Society of Nephrology. www.asn-online.org

Barnes and Noble. A brick and mortar bookstore with an online component. http://www.barnesandnoble.com

Baxter Healthcare Corporation. Highly informative site. http://www.renalinfo.com/us

Body Mass Calculator. On the U.S. Dept. of Health and Human Services' website. http://www.nhlbisupport.com/bmi/bminojs.htm

Clinical Trials.gov. This address is specifically for CKD trials. http://clinicaltrials.gov/ct2/results?term=Chronic+Kidney+Disease

DaVita. A private dialysis company which also provides kidney education, forum, recipes, tools, and blogs. http://www.davita.com

Dictionary.com. A general dictionary. http://www.dictionary.reference.com

Discovery Channel. Offers free workout videos. http://fittv.discovery.com/

Drugs.com. Explains the purpose of drugs you may be using. [You'll have to wade through commercial advertisements, though.] http://www.drugs.com

Health Central. Short articles on medical topics with links to more comprehensive information. http://www. healthcentral.com

International Diagnosis Codes, 10th Revision. http://apps.who.int/classifications/apps/icd/icd10online/

Kidney. A traditional Google search, so be prepared to be inundated with hits. http://directory.google.com/Top/Health/Conditions_and_Diseases/Genitourinary_Disorders/

Lab Tests Online. Defines lab tests and their purpose. [You may need a medical dictionary to understand what you read here.] http://www.labtestsonline.org

Libre Clothing. Clothes designed for the infusion patient. www.LibreClothing.com

Medhelp. Varied information about CKD. http://www.medhelp.org/medical-information/show/1/Chronic-renal-failure

Medical Dictionary Online. Not as comprehensive as others. http://www.online-medical-dictionary.org

Medical Education Institute Inc. Classes on a variety of kidney related topics. http://www.kidneyschool.org

Medical Education Institute Inc. Their other kidney disease education site. http://www.lifeoptions.org

Medicare & Medicaid. http://www.medicare.gov

MedicineNet.com. Dictionary, symptoms, procedures, test, medications. http://www.medicinenet.com

MedicineNet.com. Medical dictionary. http://www. medterms.com/Script/Main/hp.asp

Medline Plus. Information about herbal medicine. www.nlm.nih.gov/medlineplus/herbalmedicine.html

Medmark.org. Articles about the kidneys. http://www. medmark.org/neph

Merriam-Webster Dictionary Online. Includes a medical search option. http://www.merriam-webster.com/

National Agricultural Library's Food and Nutrition Information. http://fnic.nal.usda.gov/nal_display/index.php?tax_level=1&info_center=4

National Center for Complementary and Alternative Medicine. www.nccam.nih.gov

National Institutes of Health. Includes dietary supplements. http://www.nih.gov

National Kidney Disease Education Program. http:// nkdep.nih.gov

National Kidney Foundation. http://www.kidney.org

National Kidney and Urologic Diseases Information Clearinghouse. Permits use of content, since it is copyright free. http://www.kidney.niddk.nih.gov

National Institutes of Health and the United States National Library of Medicine's health information. You can search for caregivers, doctors or health care service, health facilities, drugs, medical dictionary and news releases from the New York Times Syndicate, the AP News Service and Reuters via this site. http://www.nlm.nih.gov/medlineplus

National Library of Medicine, Medline Plus. Information about complementary and alternative medicine. http://www.nlm.nih.gov/medlineplus/complementary andalternativemedicine.html

National Library of Medicine at the National Institutes of Health. Database of biomedical and heath care books, slides, computer software, and databases. [Unfortunately, only a handful was published after 2000.] When you find the title you want, you need to check your local library since this is not a circulation library. http://locatorplus.gov/

National Organization for Rare Diseases. http://www.rarediseases.org/search/orgsearch?org_ name=kidney+disease&SUBMIT=Submit+Query.

Nephron Information Center. http://www.nephron.com

Open Directory list of sources. People like you and me can opt to maintain or edit a section of this website. http://www.dmoz.org/Health/Medicine/Medical_ Specialties/Nephrology

Physicians' Desk Reference. You will have to register to use this site which provides drug dosage taking into account kidney function among other information. www.pdr.net

PR Newswire Association, Inc. Articles. Use the search option and remember that some of these articles may be biased since they were released by businesses in an attempt to sell their product. http://www.prnewsire. com

Renal Support Network. Articles and information at http://KidneyTimes.com. and a discussion forum at http://www.kidneyspace.com.

Reuters' Medical News. Database of daily postings of new medical issue articles. While there is a listing of arti-cles, there is also a search option. In addition to daily free articles, subscriptions are available. http://www.reutershealth.com/en/index.html

Revolutionhealth.com. More information about CKD. http://www.revolutionhealth.com/conditions/kidney-bladder/kidney-disease/?s_kwcid=kidney | 85388585-4

United States Department of Health and Human Ser-vices. Articles of interest on different aspects of dis-eases, health and nutrition. http://www.healthfinder.gov

United States Department of Health and Human Ser-vices. Dietary Guidelines for Americans [was to be updated in late 2010]. http://www.health.gov/dietary guidelines/

United States Department of Health and Human Services. FDA U.S. Food and Drug Administration. http://www.fda.gov/Food/default.htm

United States Pharmacopeia. Explanation of drugs used in scripts. http:/www.usp.org

Webmed.com. Simple, direct explanation of CKD. http://www.webmd.com/a-to-z-guides/chronic-kidney-disease-topic-overview

Yahoo. General health information about CKD. http://health.yahoo.net/search?q1=Chronic+Kidney+Disease

Yahoo. Traditional search. [Be prepared to be inundated with hits.] http://dir.yahoo.com/Health/Diseases_and_Conditions/Kidney_Diseases

CHAPTER 14

Glossary

Acanthosis nigricans: A disease that causes velvety, light-brown-to-black markings usually on the neck, under the arms or in the groin.

ACE Inhibitor: A blood pressure medication that lowers protein in the urine if you have CKD.

Acute: Extremely painful, severe or serious, quick onset, of short duration; the opposite of chronic.

Acyanosis: No blue skin from lack of oxygen.

Albumin: Water soluble protein in the blood.

Anemia: A blood disease in which the number of healthy red blood cells decreases.

Anicteric sclera: The white of the eye is not jaundiced or yellowed.

Antibiotic: Medication used to treat infection.

Arteries: Vessels that carry blood *from* the heart.

Asymptomatic: Without indications of a disease.

Auscultation: Listening to the sounds within your body, usually with a stethoscope.

Benign: Harmless - as in benign rather than malignant [life threatening] tumor.

Bid: From the Latin bis in die meaning twice a day, usually found in the directions for a script.

Bounding: Used to describe your pulse as strong and forceful.

Calcium: The electrolyte responsible for bone and teeth formation and growth, although that is only one of its jobs.

Carbohydrate: A substance in food that the body reduces to simple sugars and uses as a major energy source.

CAT scan: multiple x-rays taken by computerized axial tomography which are then combined into one picture of the inside of the body, has the advantage over an x-ray of also being able to show soft tissue damage.

CBC: A complete blood count, a comprehensive blood test.

Certification: Your doctor has taken training in his/her specialty and passed the final exam – the *board* in board certification - for the course in order to become certified in the particular specialty.

Cholesterol: While the basis for both sex hormones and bile, can cause blockages if it accumulates in the lining of a blood vessel.

Chronic: Long term, the opposite of acute.

Chronic Kidney Disease: Damage to the kidneys for more than three months, which cannot be reversed but may be slowed.

Circulatory Diseases: Those affecting the circulatory system, basically the heart, blood and blood vessels.

CKD: See Chronic Kidney Disease.

Conjunctiva: The mucous membrane that lines the inner eyelid and the exposed surface of the eyeball.

Claudication: Leg weakness associated with circulatory problems.

Creatinine clearance: Compares the creatinine level in your urine with that in your blood to provide information about your kidney function.

Cyst: An abnormal sac in the body which contains air, fluid or a semi-solid substance.

Dyslipidemia: Abnormal levels of cholesterol, triglyceride or both.

Diuretic: Usually a drug ingested to increase the output of urine.

Dyspnea: Difficulty breathing.

Dysuria: Difficult or painful urination.

Edema: Swelling caused by fluid retention in the tissues of the body.

Effusion: leaking.

Erythropoietin: Produced by the kidneys to spur red blood cell production.

Fasting: No food or drink for a specified time, usually from after midnight for blood tests.

Fatigue: Lack of energy and motivation, possibly caused by low iron levels.

Gallop: Different sounds in the heart.

Genitourinary: Dealing with the genital and urinary systems of the body.

GFR: Glomerular filtration rate [if there is a lower case "e" before the term, it means estimated glomerular filtration rate] which determines both the stage of kidney disease and how well the kidneys are functioning.

Glucose: The main sugar found in the blood. In diabetes, the body doesn't adequately control natural and ingested sugar.

HBP: The abbreviation for high blood pressure, see hypertension.

Hematuria: Blood in the urine.

Hemoglobin: Transports oxygen in the blood via red blood cells and gives the red blood cells their color.

Hemoptysis: Coughing up blood.

High Blood Pressure: See hypertension.

Hormones: Gland produced chemicals that trigger tissues to do whatever their particular job is.

Hypertension: A possible cause of CKD, 140/90 mm Hg is currently considered hypertension, a risk factor for heart disease and stroke, too.

Hypertensive nephrosclerosis: Kidney damage caused by HBP.

Hypertriglyceridemia: High triglyceride [major form of fat stored in the body] levels.

ICD: International Statistical Classification of Disease and Related Health Problems, provides the medical codes for illnesses.

Ingested: Taken by mouth.

Integumentary: The skin and its associates like the nails.

Interaction: Food or other medications which will affect how the one being prescribed works.

Kidney Stone: Stone caused in the urinary tract and kidney when crystals adhere to each other. Most of those in the kidneys are made of calcium.

Lab: Short hand for medical laboratory, the place where your biological specimens are drawn and analyzed to ascertain the state of your health [think blood and urine, usually].

Lymphadenopathy: Disease of the lymph nodes.

M.A.: Short hand for medical assistant, the one who helps your health practitioner with clinical and administrative matters in the office.

Medicaid: U.S. government health insurance for those with limited income.

Medicare: U.S. government health insurance for those over 65, those having certain special needs, or those who have end stage renal disease.

Meds: Short hand for medication, chemical substances in the form of a script to treat, cure, or prevent disease.

Melena: Black, tarry, bloody stool.

MRI: Magnetic Resonance Imaging - a non-invasive method of imagining [seeing] the inside of your body.

Nausea: The feeling in the upper stomach that you need to vomit or are queasy.

Nephrolithiasis: Kidney stones.

Nephrologist: Renal or kidney and hypertension specialist.

Nephrology: The subspecialty of internal medicine which deals with the kidneys and hypertension.

Nephrons: The part of the kidney that actually purifies and filters the blood.

Nephropathy: Kidney disease.

Nondistended: Not swollen.

NSAID: Non-steroidal anti-inflammatory drugs such as ibuprofen, aspirin, Aleve or naproxen usually used for arthritis or pain management, can worsen kidney disease, sometimes irreversibly.

Oral thrush: A mouth disease that can occur in people with compromised immune systems.

Orthostatis: Fall in blood pressure which produces dizziness upon standing.

Oxalate: A simple molecule found in foods which sometimes combines with calcium to form kidney stones.

P.A.: Short hand for physician's assistant, someone who is licensed to practice medicine under a licensed doctor's supervision.

Paroxysmal nocturnal dyspnea: Sudden, recurring night bouts of shortness of breath.

Phosphorus: One of the electrolytes, works with calcium for bone formation, but too much can cause calcification where you don't want it: joints, eyes, skin and heart.

Po: From the Latin per os meaning by mouth, usually found in the directions for a script.

Potassium: One of the electrolytes, important because it counteracts sodium's effect on blood pressure.

Protein: Amino acids arranged in chains joined by peptide bonds to form a compound, important because some proteins are hormones, enzymes and antibodies.

Proteinuria: Protein in the urine, not a normal state of being.

Purine: Compound found mainly in beef, poultry, pork and fish that is metabolized into uric acid.

Pruritus: Itching, one whose cause might be kidney disease.

Rales: Crackling, clicking or rattling sounds in the lungs.

Renal: Of or about the kidneys.

Renin: Hormone that regulates blood pressure.

Rhonchi: Dry, leathery sounds in the lungs.

Script: Short hand for lab work order or prescription [orders from a medical practitioner for a pharmacy to provide medication or a medical device] depending upon how the term is used.

Sphygmomanometer: The cuff, the measuring device and the wires that connect the two in a machine used to measure your blood pressure, commonly called a blood pressure meter.

T3: Part of the CBC which measures your triiodothyronine, which is a thyroid hormone that plays an important role in controlling your metabolism. If the T3 reading is abnormal, then the T4 test is ordered to find out what the problem might be.

Tid: From the Latin ter in die meaning three times a day, usually found in the directions for a script.

Ultrasound: A certain kind of X ray that requires no radiation.

Ureter: Carries urine from the kidneys to the bladder.

Veins: Vessels that carry blood *toward* the heart.

Vitamin D: Regulates calcium and phosphorous blood levels as well as promoting bone formation, among other tasks - affects the immune system.

Bibliography

Alexander, Ivy L. *Urinary Tract And Kidney Diseases And Disorders Sourcebook Basic Consumer Health Information About the Urinary System, Including the Bladder, Urethra, ... Reference Series)* Detroit: Omnigraphics, Inc., 2005. Print.

American College of Physicians and Reliant Pharmaceuticals. "An ACP Special Report: Understanding and Managing Your Triglycerides." Greensboro: The Stay Well Company, 2006. Print.

American Society of Nephrology, The. "Kidney Disease: A Serious Threat to Public Health." Web. 13 Aug. 2010

Auer, Juliet et al. *Living Well with Kidney Failure.* Grand Rapids: Class Pub., 2004. Print

"Basic Chemistry Profile." BioHealth Diagnostics. Web. 7 Sept. 2009.

Castle, Erik. "Low-phosphorus diet: Best for kidney disease? - MayoClinic.com." Mayo Clinic medical information and tools for healthy living - MayoClinic.com. Web. 13 July 2009.

Curtis, Judith, A. *Renal Patient's Guide to Good Eating: a Cookbook for Patients by a Patient.* Springfield: C.C. Thomas, 1989. Print.

"Glomerulus." Gale Encyclopedia of Medicine. Farmington Hills: Thomson Gale, 2008. Print.

"Kidney and Urologic Diseases Statistics for the United States." National Kidney and Urologic Diseases Information Clearinghouse. Web. 28 June 2009.

Koble, Nina. *Ten Step Diet & Lifestyle Plan for Healthier Kidneys: Avoid Dialysis.* St. Louis: Mirasmart Digital Pub., 2009. Print

Mattern, Joanne. *Unlocking the Secrets of Science: Profiling 20th Century Achievers in Science, Medicine, and Technology – Joseph E. Murray and the Story of the First Human Kidney Transplant.* Hockessin: Mitchell Lane Pub., 2003. Print.

"Milestones." *Time* 13 July 2009: 21. Print.

O'Callaghan, Christopher A., and Barry Brenner. *The Kidney at a Glance.* Grand Rapids: Blackwell, Inc., 2000. Print.

Parker, James N., and Icon Health Publications. *The 2002 Official Patient's Sourcebook on Kidney Failure.* Minneapolis: ICON Health Pub., 2002. Print.

Riley, Jess. *Driving Sideways.* New York: Ballantine Books, 2008. Print.

Seidick, Kathryn. *Or you can let him go.* New York: Delacorte, 1984. Print.

Stein, Andy, and Janet Wild. *Kidney Failure Explained* Grand Rapids: Class, 2002. Print.

Tracy, Kathleen. *Unlocking the Secrets of Science: Profiling 20th Century Achievers in Science, Medicine, and Technology – Willem Kolff and the Invention of the Dialysis Machine.* Hockessin: Mitchell Lane Pub., 2003. Print.

Townsend, Raymond R. MD. and Debbie L. Cohen MD. *100 Questions & Answers about Kidney Disease and Hypertension.* Sudbury: Jones and Bartlett Pub., 2009.

"Urinalysis." The University of Utah. Spencer S. Eccles Health Science Library. Web. 7 Sept. 2009.

Walser, Mackenzie, and Betsy Thorpe. *Coping with Kidney Disease: A 12-Step Treatment Program to Help You Avoid Dialysis.* New York: Wiley, 2004. Print.

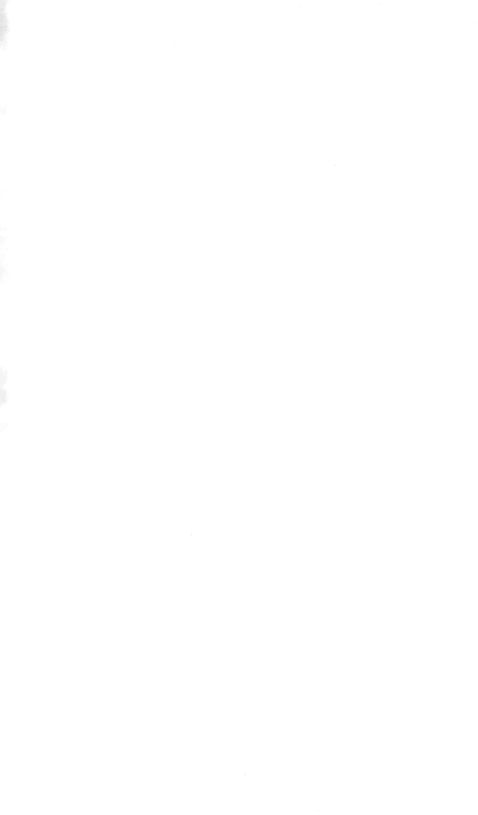

CPSIA information can be obtained
at www.ICGtesting.com
Printed in the USA
BVHW030330260719
554329BV00002B/273/P

9 781457 502149